"This text is a great how-to resource for supervisors who aspire to ensure high quality services and experiences for their clients and behavior technicians. Silbaugh provides an easy-to-follow framework by which practitioners can systematically monitor and evaluate behavioral objectives and teaching procedures by incorporating both measures of fidelity and interobserver agreement. Data collection guidelines and questions are presented along with practical examples and tips for overcoming common obstacles. A must use for early career analysts or seasoned clinicians looking to support claims of high-quality services!"

Ivy Chong, *PhD, BCBA-D, Chief Clinical Officer, Little Leaves Behavioral Services, Mid Atlantic and Florida, USA*

Quality Control for Behavior Analysts

Quality Control for Behavior Analysts helps practitioners apply concepts of quality planning, control, and improvement to implement high-quality behavioral interventions that maximize care value through superior clinical outcomes.

Unlock the secrets of delivering high-quality behavioral interventions with this indispensable handbook designed for the Board Certified Behavior Analyst (BCBA®). Starting with an introductory overview and concise history of quality, this book demystifies key concepts like quality assurance, planning, control, and improvement for the practicing BCBA and other stakeholders in the applied behavior analysis (ABA) autism service industry. Discover how behavior analysts can apply these concepts to effectively manage the quality of their behavioral interventions through the frequent routine assessment of procedural fidelity and interobserver agreement during ABA therapy. With its practical guidance and step-by-step approach, this book empowers BCBAs to effectively control the quality of their interventions in the evidence-based practice of ABA in ways that can dramatically improve care value and the quality of life for people with autism. This guide is a vital resource for any BCBA committed to providing high-quality ABA therapy and making a difference in the lives of individuals with autism.

Bryant C. Silbaugh, PhD, BCBA, LBA, is a former assistant professor of special education, founder of the National ABA Service Quality Network, and an internationally recognized behavior analyst specializing in the behavioral assessment and treatment of autism spectrum disorder.

Quality Control for Behavior Analysts

How to Manage Behavioral Intervention Quality in Autism Service Settings

Bryant C. Silbaugh

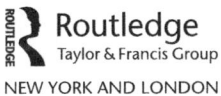

Routledge
Taylor & Francis Group

NEW YORK AND LONDON

First published 2025
by Routledge
605 Third Avenue, New York, NY 10158

and by Routledge
4 Park Square, Milton Park, Abingdon, Oxon, OX14 4RN

Routledge is an imprint of the Taylor & Francis Group, an informa business

© 2025 Bryant C. Silbaugh

ISBN: 978-1-032-75384-3 (hbk)
ISBN: 978-1-032-75666-0 (pbk)
ISBN: 978-1-003-47509-5 (ebk)

DOI: 10.4324/9781003475095

Typeset in Times New Roman
by Apex CoVantage, LLC

This book is dedicated to the memory of Dr. Jose Martinez-Diaz, a man whose compassion for practitioners of applied behavior analysis (ABA) and dedication to the quality of ABA teaching and service delivery were unmatched.

Contents

Preface

It was the spring of 2020, at the onset of the COVID-19 pandemic. I was approaching the end of my third year as a tenure-track Assistant Professor of Special Education at the University of Texas at San Antonio (UTSA). I had just initiated a new line of research with Dr. Robbie El Fattal, Chief Executive Officer and Co-Founder of Cultivate Behavioral Health, focused on the quality of applied behavior analysis (ABA) autism service delivery. I was up for review with my department and the Dean. Unfortunately, the Dean decided I would not be offered an extension of my contract to a 4th year, which meant that I was no longer considered for tenure. I was afraid of what would be next for me because of all the uncertainty that the pandemic brought to our lives, but I decided that my best move was to resign. At the end of the spring semester, I left UTSA and returned to the ABA autism clinical service industry full-time in San Antonio.

There's a longer story there, but what really captured my attention upon my return to full-time work in clinical ABA settings were the many barriers that prevented practitioners from regularly assessing procedural fidelity and interobserver agreement in behavioral intervention. As a researcher, I understood how absolutely vital it is to first verify the conditions under which your behavioral data are collected, and the quality of those data, before visually analyzing graphed data and making clinical decisions based on those data. If you have bad data, you will make bad decisions. Plain and simple! And I think the practitioners I met knew that too. As W. Edwards Deming is famous for saying, "A bad system will beat a good person, every time". I don't know if that's true, but I do know that bad systems are everywhere. I thought that if I was going to immerse myself in clinical work, and potentially expose myself to bad systems, I would have to develop new, practical, and efficient methods for assessing procedural fidelity and interobserver agreement that any Board Certified Behavior Analyst (BCBA®) could use for any behavioral intervention, anywhere, any time.

A year later, I was fortunate to meet Jennifer Alaniz, a clinical BCBA, and her husband David Yassa, founders and owners of New Beginnings Academy. Jennifer liked my published work on the ABA service delivery quality

(ASDQ) framework, and we immediately connected on our passion for doing what it takes to build an ABA autism service organization committed to high-quality service delivery. Over the next year as a clinical supervisor, and then as Director of Clinical Quality, I had the pleasure of working with Jennifer and David and a number of other wonderful practitioners to develop the current model of behavioral intervention quality (BIQ). I also had the honor of collaborating with Dr. Jon Bailey, whose interest was piqued by the ASDQ framework, and generously provided me with the mentorship I needed to present the current quality control model at conferences and write about it in this book in a way that the everyday BCBA supervisor can relate to. I am forever in these colleagues' debt.

During the year that I developed the current model, I interviewed a number of Registered Behavior Technicians (RBT®s) and BCBAs for positions available at our company. For most of the applicants, I asked them either to define procedural fidelity or interobserver agreement, or to explain how they would assess procedural fidelity and interobserver agreement if they worked at New Beginnings Academy. Can you guess what percentage of the candidates answered these questions satisfactorily? When I asked this question to an audience at the annual convention of the Florida Association for Behavior Analysis, the audience guessed 0–30%, depending on the question. They were very close! To my memory, none of the candidates I interviewed could answer those questions. Does that mean they were bad clinicians? Absolutely not. But it did tell me those candidates worked in environments that failed to reinforce verbal behavior about procedural fidelity and interobserver agreement and I worried their implementation of these best practice assessments may not have been reinforced either. The Florida conference audience was the first to hear me present on the current model. To get the audience warmed up and ready for what I was about to present, I told them about an important experience I had at work just two days prior to the conference.

The conference was on a Thursday, and that Tuesday I visited the home of a new client referred to our company for ABA services. He was a 3-year-old boy with autism spectrum disorder and I was visiting him and his mother at home to conduct a direct assessment of his verbal behavior and social skills with the Verbal Behavior Milestones Assessment and Placement Program (VB-MAPP®). What I found was a boy who could not talk, imitate, follow basic 1-step instructions, or follow gestures. I asked his mother if she could select a few toys he likes to play with so I could observe their interactions. She walked through the kitchen to her room in the back of the house and the boy stayed with me in the living room, so I took the opportunity to build some rapport.

I smiled, and I said some of the same playful things I would say to my own 3-year-old son to get a smile. I pretended to hide behind objects in the room, and I pretended to approach and tickle him. That was the moment he looked at me, walked to me, and held up his arms. I quickly scooped him up, smiled, held him in my arms, and said emphatically, "hello!". He laid his head on my shoulder as if we already met. After we walked around the room a bit and I talked about what I saw (e.g., "Ooh, look at that big TV!"), I tried to set him down. Only, he clung to me like I was dropping him off a cliff. I set him down, and he looked up at me with terror in his eyes, crying, screaming, reaching up at me, until I scooped him up again in my arms. He laid his head on my shoulder and he was at peace. I tried to set him down a few more times and he gave the same reaction. I realized that I was not going to put him down until he was ready or until something else motivating in his environment caught his attention. And then for a moment, as I held him in my arms, he felt familiar.

He felt just like my son. He felt the same way my own son felt in my arms as I hugged him, rocked him, and put him to bed every night. And I was reminded that the quality of care we provide to this boy and his family must be equal to or greater than the quality of care I would expect for my own son. I thought to myself at that very moment that I was so glad we found him. We can help him. We have to help him. In a few weeks, I am going to send my team to his home and we are going to have to design effective behavioral interventions to help him. But our interventions will not work if we do not implement them with high procedural fidelity and interobserver agreement. I refuse to personally implement and/or supervise behavioral interventions without quality control. I was sad because my experience told me that this child's journey was not going to be an easy one, but I was optimistic at the same time. Because for the past year we had developed a robust model of quality control over BIQ that I was confident I could put into place for as long as we provide him with ABA services, which would ensure that the interventions I design would be implemented with a high degree of accuracy and consistency.

If you have picked up this book, there is a good chance that you have been in situations just like this one. And with the model described herein, I know you too can deliver behavioral interventions with high procedural fidelity and interobserver agreement. Frequently engaging in quality control over our behavioral interventions is the right thing to do. If you put the methods in this book into practice, I hope you will consider e mailing me to share your story and your journey to delivering high-quality behavioral interventions in ABA autism service delivery with quality planning, quality control, and quality improvement.

Acknowledgements

I don't know if I would have had the courage to write this book without the encouragement of Jon Bailey. I first met Jon when he took an interest in the ASDQ framework and reached out to me and my colleague to discuss our ideas about quality. The year thereafter he was kind enough to mentor me and teach me how to design and deliver presentations at conferences that resonate with the everyday BCBA clinical supervisor. It was through that experience I learned to communicate the science and practice of ABA in more relatable ways without overwhelming an audience with too much information. I did my best to generalize that skill to writing this book.

I certainly would not have written this book were it not for the intellectual and creative freedom afforded to me by Jennifer Alaniz and her husband David Yassa, my employers, colleagues, and friends at New Beginnings Academy. Jennifer and David trusted my vision for quality control over behavioral interventions and supported my efforts to develop the model every step of the way. I will forever be grateful to them.

I also need to thank some of the RBTs who were there at the beginning and continue to endorse its utility, and therefore played a major role in its development. Thank you Kimberly Edvalson, Briana Lawson, Laycia Robinson, and Natasha Tsandoula. I'm forever grateful for their commitment to quality!

I'm thankful also for Dr. Robbie El Fattal for believing in my abilities years ago and inspiring me to pursue research on quality. I may never have gone in this direction had he not asked me one day, during a consultation, how to determine if an organization provided high-quality services. I said I had no idea and that we should study it. The rest is history.

Lastly, I thank my wife, Dorothy Silbaugh, for believing in my ability to write books in this field that can help people.

Introduction

Clinical behavior analysts who serve individuals with autism and other developmental disorders work in a wide variety of extremely complicated settings, in the face of many barriers. To get the job done well, a clinical behavior analyst need tools, methods, processes, and so forth that are extremely practical, efficient, and generalizable. Accordingly, my primary goal in writing this book was to help clinical behavior analysts practicing in ABA autism service settings acquire foundational quality knowledge that they can use to control the quality of their behavioral interventions; no matter who they are, where they work, who their clients are, what interventions they design, who their RBTs are, regardless of whether they are supported by their organization's infrastructure, whether they work as a lone wolf in homes and communities or alongside fellow clinicians in a treatment facility, and so on. In other words, no matter what the circumstances are, a behavior analyst who can program effective interventions can ensure that those interventions will be implemented correctly and yield the data that they need to get the job done well. My secondary goal in writing this book was to inspire a variety of stakeholders within the ABA autism service industry to support the efforts of aspiring and current clinical behavior analysts to promote quality assurance in their organizations and the field broadly with quality control over behavioral interventions.

How to Use This Book

If you are a clinical BCBA supervisor, I hope you picked up this book to learn how to control the quality of your behavioral interventions. If that is the case, use Chapter 1 to learn some vocabulary and basic concepts pertaining to quality, with a focus on the quality trilogy: quality planning, quality control, and quality improvement. You will directly apply those concepts in the next chapter. The other concepts such as ISO 9001 and the ASDQ framework are less relevant to you as a reader but could help you expand your thinking to process systems-level ideas about quality assurance that will become more important later in your career if you are in the position to manage quality control processes implemented by other clinical BCBA supervisors. If you are a clinical director at an ABA autism service organization or hold a similar position, everything in this chapter is applicable to you, especially the ASDQ framework; description, prediction, and control over ASDQ; and the elements of quality assurance systems in human service settings. You will apply these ideas in Chapter 4 as a manager for quality.

In Chapter 2, clinical BCBA supervisors and clinical directors should carefully read all of the content page by page, and follow the prompts to develop a quality plan. Note that in this context, the term "quality plan" refers to a plan to conduct quality control cycles in practice. In later chapters, a "quality plan" refers to a behavioral intervention protocol, or how the RBT should intervene on the target behavior.

Chapter 3 guides clinical BCBAs through the implementation of their quality plan to start controlling quality with quality control cycles. Clinical directors who have been inspired to support clinical behavior analysts' use of the current model should have mastered implementation of the current model themselves before attempting to manage others' implementation of quality control cycles. Accordingly, after putting this chapter to use to master the model themselves, clinical directors should periodically revisit this chapter in their support for other clinical BCBA supervisors implementing the model for the first time.

Chapter 4 was written primarily for clinical directors. Clinical directors should read this chapter to develop their quality plan for managing BIQ indirectly through the clinical BCBA supervisors who report to them. Clinical BCBA supervisors will find this chapter useful for understanding the broader context within which they may be implementing quality control cycles, and the contingencies clinical directors can arrange to ensure that clinical BCBA control over BIQ is reinforced and maintained over time. However, if their goal is just to get straight to the business of implementing quality control cycles, clinical BCBA supervisors are advised to skim this chapter and perhaps even skip everything after the section on controlling cultural practices with quality management. Researchers and clinical directors interested in conducting research on the variables that influence dimensions of quality control cycles and their outcomes will find the latter half of this chapter perhaps much more relevant.

Clinical BCBA supervisors and clinical directors should read Chapter 5 in its entirety if they are still on the fence about whether the current model of quality control will be beneficial to their practice, and have not implemented the model yet. However, if any of the readers has already started to implement quality control cycles and are already seeing the benefits, they can skip this chapter altogether and move to Chapter 6 for troubleshooting.

If you arrive at Chapter 6 before you implement quality control cycles, consider this chapter a guide to proactively prevent potential problems that could arise when you get started. Alternatively, anyone reading this book who has started to implement quality control cycles should frequently revisit this chapter to strategically troubleshoot as barriers arise. If a reader encounters barriers that are not addressed in Chapter 6, I hope that they will e mail me and share their experience. Maybe, we can solve the problem together!

Anyone reading this book should save Chapter 7 for last. If you are a clinical BCBA supervisor or clinical director currently implementing quality control cycles, hold off on reading this chapter until you have mastered the model. Once you have mastered the model, this chapter will offer you advice on what to do next along your new quality assurance journey in your organization and the ABA autism service industry broadly. If you are anyone else reading this book, this chapter offers advice on how to support clinicians and organizations in the adoption of the current model.

1 Quality Concepts and Definitions

"[quality]. . . is something fundamental that cultures do. It's all about planning to do something, doing that something, noticing the variability and trying to continuously improve to reduce the variability of whatever it is you're doing, and then trying to take it to the next level."

—*Building Better Businesses in ABA Podcast*

Let the year 2024 be remembered as the year the applied behavior analysis (ABA) autism service industry started to take the quality of their behavioral interventions seriously. In 1968, the founding fathers of the field of applied behavior analysis defined ABA in terms of seven dimensions (Baer et al., 1968). Applied behavior analysis was to be applied, behavioral, analytic, effective, conceptually systematic, generalizable, and technological. When interventions are applied, their social significance is apparent. Interventions are behavioral when the target of the intervention is an aspect of the learner's behavior, not the behavior of the people around them or hypothetical constructs such as traits or states. Interventions are analytic when practitioners conduct systematic treatment evaluations to demonstrate that behavior change is really the result of the intervention. When learner behavior improves in large, meaningful ways, an intervention is effective. Conceptually systematic behavioral interventions describe and explain behavior and its determinants in terms of fundamental principles of behavior. To the extent that improvements in behavior are apparent in untrained contexts and maintain over time, behavioral interventions have generality. In order to implement behavioral interventions in accordance with those dimensions, their descriptions must be sufficiently objective, clear, precise, and complete to enable a change agent to implement the intervention accurately. In other words, they must be what Baer and colleagues (1968) called "technological". When interventions are accurately implemented, practitioners have the opportunity to evaluate the extent to which all the other dimensions of ABA are met over time.

Today, most behavioral interventions are delivered by someone other than the behavior analysts who designed them. For example, in the most prevalent

DOI: 10.4324/9781003475095-1

of ABA service models in the autism service industry, a Board Certified Behavior Analyst (BCBA®) designs and supervises behavioral interventions implemented largely by a behavioral technician or Registered Behavior Technician (RBT®) and other stakeholders such as parents, childcare providers, or paraprofessionals in special education. When the technological dimension is met, behavior technicians and other stakeholders can implement them with accuracy, but only under conditions in which reinforcing contingencies for accurately implementing behavioral intervention plans are present. But how do practitioners evaluate the extent to which the technological dimension of a behavioral intervention is met? And what are the contingencies under which this practice can be maintained in everyday service delivery settings? This book will answer both of these questions and enable you to immediately start addressing these issues and elevating the quality of the services you provide.

I argue that a behavioral intervention meets the technological dimension to the extent that a change agent can implement the intervention and collect data on the learner's response to intervention with sufficient accuracy to enable data-based decisions that improve the response to intervention. ABA researchers have developed two general assessments for this purpose: procedural fidelity and interobserver agreement (Cooper et al., 2020). Procedural fidelity assessments are used to evaluate the extent to which a behavioral intervention is planned. This type of assessment answers questions such as "Did the change agent use the same discriminative stimuli, prompt fading procedure, and schedule of reinforcement specified by the intervention protocol?" Interobserver agreement assessments are used to evaluate the believability of behavior data. Two observers independently observe the intervention implemented and collect data on the learner's behavior. At the end of the observation the observers compare their data and calculate the extent to which their data agree. High agreement equals high believability. This assessment answers questions such as "Do we believe those data and can we use those data to make appropriate treatment decisions?"

For over 50 years since the founding fathers conceptualized the technological dimension of ABA, behavior analysts in research and practice settings have used procedural fidelity and interobserver agreement assessments to evaluate the technological dimension of their interventions. But researchers historically have failed to report procedural fidelity in their studies consistently (St. Peter et al., 2023), and practical methods for overcoming barriers to the daily use of procedural fidelity and interobserver agreement assessments by behavior analysts and change agents are lacking and in very high demand (Morris et al., 2022, 2024). Moreover, ABA research on the process of implementing these assessments in practice, and the variables in practice settings that influence practitioners' implementation of these assessments is largely absent.

I do not think we need to wait for ABA researchers to catch up. In this book, I will describe a highly efficient and practical model that behavior analysts can use anytime, anywhere, with any protocol, and any client, to rapidly assess the technological dimension of their intervention, improve procedural fidelity and interobserver agreement, arrange contingencies that support behavior analysts' routine use of these practices, and enable systematic evaluations of supervision effectiveness that result in consistently high-quality behavioral interventions.

Robust industry-wide quality control over behavioral interventions is a vital step in the future of quality in the ABA autism service industry. By reflecting on the history of quality broadly, apparent similarities between the evolution of quality management practices and the development of quality assurance in the ABA autism service delivery, begin to emerge. And by understanding those similarities, we are perhaps better equipped to predict our future and act more effectively with respect to ensuring that the future is bright.

Quality in Ancient China

The noun "Quality" can be traced back to the 14th century and comes from the Latin *qualitas* (Merriam-Webster.com, 2023). But managing for quality has been traced back thousands of years (Qiupeng et al., 1995). If you were a Chinese pottery maker sometime between the 16th- and 11th-century BCE China, you would make some of the highest quality pottery in the world. That is because the Shang Dynasty of China dominated the world roughly 3,600 years ago, in the manufacturing of goods such as pottery, leather, textile, architecture, and ship building. They accomplished their reputation for quality through centralized organizations that exerted quality control over the handicraft industry through specialized functions that resemble how quality is managed today: the regulation of materials, manufacturing, finished product storage and distribution, standards set for quality and productivity, and product inspecting and testing in relation to standards (Qiupeng et al., 1995).

Quality in Medieval Europe

Now fast forward to the 21st-century quality movement. How quality looks today has its roots in the medieval European guilds of the late 13th century (American Society for Quality; ASQ, n.d.). You are still a pottery maker and you still produce a very high-quality product, but that is because the personal stakes you, as a craftsman, have in maintaining customer satisfaction, are very high. You sell all your products locally, so your reputation is important, and you cannot afford to lose customers. Word-of-mouth is almost exclusively how you ensure repeat business, so you cannot afford to sell faulty goods. For quality assurance, you mark all of your goods with a craftsman mark to track any faulty goods in case some got past your own inspection or quality control, and so that future customers know who to go to for more high-quality pottery. You and several other pottery makers form a union, known at the time as a guild, and work together to develop rules for product and service quality and maintain standards for products and services. Your guild forms a committee to enforce those rules by marking the highest-quality pottery with the guild's mark or symbol. Your own mark, like the logo of an ABA autism service organization today, in combination with the mark of the guild, analogous to the logo of an accrediting body that accredits organizations based on quality, symbolize your reputation and function as quality assurance. This approach to quality assurance in manufacturing was predominant until things changed with the emergence of the factory system in Great Brittan in the mid-18th century and the Industrial Revolution.

Quality in the Factory System

During the Industrial Revolution, the European factory system led to specialization, with quality maintained through skilled labor and inspections. In the factory system, you and other craftsmen like you would likely become specialists who work for shop owners. The shop owners would function as production supervisors responsible for quality control and assurance. Through product inspection and audits, any defective products would be either improved or tossed out. As a result of this system, you would experience a loss of pride in your work and a sense that you have lost your autonomy.

Quality in the Taylor System of Scientific Management

The US diverged from the European factory system in the late 19th century by adopting the system developed by scientific management giant Frederick Winslow Taylor (ASQ, n.d.). Taylor believed that "the best management is a true science, resting upon clearly defined laws, rules, and principles, as a foundation" (Taylor, 1911, p. iv). And that a scientific approach to management could increase the productivity of existing workers without increasing the number of skilled workers. Essentially, Taylor suggested that we resist the urge to search for top talent and instead use scientific management to turn existing talent into top talent. It sounds to me like Taylor would have been a great behavior analyst! In application, the Taylor system increased industrial productivity with engineers who specialized in planning, and having craftsmen and supervisors execute the engineer's plans. This is similar to how organizational behavior managers in ABA autism service organizations engineer systems and processes for services delivered by autism care teams, and behavior analysts engineer behavioral interventions executed by behavior technicians. Just as the two-tiered model of behavior technicians implementing plans developed and overseen by behavior analysts has increased access to services (i.e., productivity in ABA) but not necessarily service quality (Silbaugh, 2024), the Taylor approach to industrial manufacturing led to major increases in productivity, but adversely impacted quality (ASQ, n.d.). As a result, whole inspection departments were developed to prevent defective goods from reaching customers. The increasing number of roles in ABA autism service organizations with "quality" in their title suggests that our industry may be headed toward the same.

Japan and Methodological Advancements

World War II (WWII) brought the importance of quality in military production to the fore, with extensive inspections to ensure safety (ASQ, n.d.). Initially, the US military inspected each unit of military equipment to ensure its safety, but extensive inspections required an extensive workforce. Difficulties in maintaining inspection personnel led to the US military adopting sampling inspection, using statistical control techniques developed by quality pioneer Walter Shewhart. An advantage of sampling inspection was that not every unit had to be inspected to control quality. Similarly, in this book, you will learn an innovation in quality control over behavioral intervention you can use to control the quality of your interventions without assessing procedural fidelity and interobserver agreement for every behavioral protocol.

In 1946, the ASQ was formed and the early 20th century saw a shift towards controlling processes as part of quality practices, as initiated by Walter Shewhart (ASQ, n.d.). His focus on data analysis through statistical techniques established the foundation for control charts, a modern quality tool. This was promoted by W. Edwards Deming, another key figure in the quality movement. The total quality movement in the US was a response to Japan's quality revolution post-WWII. Initially known for poor quality, Japan's focus on total quality through process improvement and people involvement led to a dramatic rise in the quality of its exports. Americans Deming and Joseph M. Juran played significant roles in this transformation, with Juran accurately predicting Japan's quality overtaking the US by the mid-1970s. The US corporations ultimately realized that they could not compete with Japanese manufacturing on price by making their products cheaper and placing limitations on imports, and a new Total Quality Management approach was adopted so corporations could compete on quality (ASQ, n.d.).

Other methodological innovations that ultimately helped close the quality gap between manufacturing in Japan and the US include Just in Time (JIT), Six Sigma developed by Motorola, DMAIC, Lean Six Sigma, Pland-Do-Check-Act, and other methods of continuous improvement, and more recently the concept of Quality 4.0—the adoption of advances in technology such as analytics and artificial intelligence to enhance quality (Juran, 2019). Readers interested in learning more about methodological advancements in quality might enjoy diving into the work of other major quality figures as well, including Armand V. Feigenbaum, Shigeo Shingo, Philip Crosby, Genichi Taguchi, and Kaoru Ishikawa (Juran, 2019).

ISO 9001

These and many other events ultimately led to the development of ISO 9001, an "international quality management system (QMS) standard" (Cochran, 2015, p. 1). This standard represents "fundamental management and quality assurance practices that can be applied by any organization". The practices include quality planning, control, and improvement; grounded in seven foundational principles of quality management: (1) customer focus, (2) leadership, (3) engagement of people, (4) process approach, (5) improvement, (6) evidence-based decision making, and (7) relationship management (Cochran, 2015, p. 2), all of which align nicely with modern ABA service delivery best practices. Detailed descriptions of these principles and their implications for total quality management can be obtained freely online from the International Organization for Standardization (ISO, 2015). As of the writing of this handbook, their website boasts there are "more than one million certificates issued to organizations in 189 countries" and "ISO 9001 is the most widely used quality management standard in the world" (ISO, n.d.). In 2015, ISO 9001:2015 was released and comes closer to a total quality approach (Juran, 2019).

ABA Service Delivery Quality

As I said about quality to Jonathan Mueller in episode 69 of his Building Better Businesses in ABA Podcast, "because it may be something fundamental and it's been around for thousands of years, there's been so many different ways to talk about it, that defining it hasn't been hard for behavior analysts. It's been hard for everybody" (Mueller, 2023). Until 2021, the concept of quality and the use of the term in relation to ABA autism services was undefined. To address this gap in the field of ABA and advance an empirical understanding of ABA service quality, Silbaugh and El Fattal (2022) defined quality at the organizational level as "the extent to which an organization's ABA products, services, and outcomes meet standards determined by professionals and consumers, over time, in response to changes in a receiving system, while maximizing the financial health of the organization".

With this definition, the authors described an ABA service delivery quality (ASDQ) framework integrating Organizational Behavior Management (OBM) and Culturo-Behavioral Science concepts that organizations can use to develop a quality assurance system capable of consistently delivering objectively verifiable high-quality ABA services. Maraca Learning in Boise, Idaho in 2022; The Place for Children with Autism, Illinois, in 2023; and New Beginnings Academy in San Antonio, Texas, in 2023; were three of the initial ABA autism service organizations to go public about using the ASDQ framework for quality assurance.

The ASDQ Framework

In an ASDQ framework, an ABA autism service organization deals with the wide variation in ABA autism service standards available to them by developing internal standards and adopting existing external standards (financial, professional, and consumer) that align with the organization's mission, vision, values, and the community they serve; which include clinical outcome standards and standards for how to achieve desired clinical outcomes. There are multiple sources of standards available to ABA autism service organizations such as the Behavioral Health Center of Excellence (BHCOE®), Council of Autism Service Providers (CASP®) and the Autism Commission on Quality (ACQ®), and the International Consortium for Health Outcomes Measurement (ICHOM®); and organizations can choose to draw from all of them.

ABA autism service organizations can adopt one standard at a time—there is no need to set them all at once. With a standard in place, an organization can focus on a specific process pertaining to the standard that impacts ASDQ. They can adopt key performance indicators to monitor the process. And based on the data, establish benchmarks for the level of performance or results associated with that process. Then they can use progress monitoring to assess benchmark attainment over time with quality control (Silbaugh, 2024).

The Purpose and Value of ABA Autism Services

ABA autism organizations exist to produce lasting improvements in the quality of the lives of their clients through behavior change. For individuals with autism, that means helping people live fulfilling self-determined lives by remediating developmental and adaptive behavior delays and deficits associated with autism and co-morbid conditions. Improvements in quality of life in ABA therapy are determined by proximal and distal outcome measures of behavior change. Proximal outcomes (i.e., short-term goals) are indicated by the mastery of behavior change targets corresponding to goals listed in treatment plans based on assessments (i.e., distal or long-term outcome measures) at the reassessment of the individual with autism at the end of an autism care cycle. The typical autism care cycle authorized by insurance companies is six months. The most common tiered ABA autism services model is based on the assumption that differences in scores between an initial assessment and subsequent re-assessment using outcome measurement instruments (e.g., Vineland Adaptive Behavior Scales III®) are the result of behavior change produced by behavioral interventions delivered by behavior technicians or RBTs who are supervised by BCBAs in the evidence-based practice of ABA (Slocum et al., 2014). Accordingly, the quality of a behavioral intervention is a vital determinant of the relationship between behavior change and long-term clinical outcomes. Behavioral intervention quality is affected by a myriad of variables as discussed extensively in this book, and of those variables, how ABA autism service organizations are paid for their services is one of the most influential. The methods described in this book can help behavior analysts control BIQ even when financial contingencies under which an organization operates, compete with clinical quality.

Current trends suggest that the ABA autism service industry may be gradually transitioning from a fee-for-service model to a value-based care (Porter & Twisberg, 2006) model in which the reimbursement for services from insurance companies will depend not on units of services delivered, but on the value of autism care. Figure 1.1 illustrates the idea that the value of autism care from an ABA service provider depends on the ratio of outcomes (and patient experience) to the cost to produce those outcomes. And those outcomes depend on the dosage of ABA recommended, the extent to which that dosage was delivered (i.e., utilization), and the quality of services delivered at that dosage. Based on those assumptions, it stands to reason that the quality of behavioral interventions is one of the most important aspects of ABA therapy to consider in the development of a quality assurance system intended to consistently deliver high-quality ABA therapy to individuals with autism. Accordingly, quality control of behavioral interventions is a foundational first step every ABA autism service organization should take in the development of a quality assurance system with the ASDQ framework. Especially, organizations that want to be competitive in a value-based reimbursement model of the future that will very likely be selective for quality indicators such as organization-wide metrics on procedural fidelity and interobserver agreement.

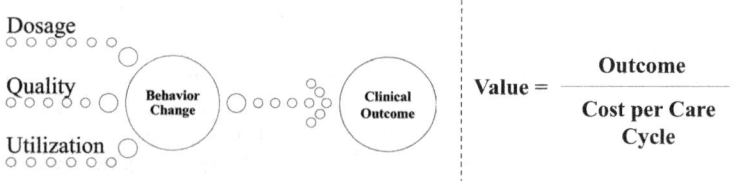

Figure 1.1 The Relationship Between Treatment, Behavior Change, Clinical Outcomes, and Care Value.

Note: Increases in the ratio of clinical outcomes to cost per care cycle for the patient correspond to increases in care value. Clinical outcomes in ABA autism service delivery are the result of behavior changes produced by behavioral interventions in the evidence-based practice of ABA. The extent of behavior change depends, among other things, on the dosage (i.e., hours) of ABA therapy prescribed, the proportion of that dosage delivered, and the quality of the behavioral interventions implemented during ABA therapy.

Describe, Predict, and Control ASDQ

High-quality evidence-based behavioral intervention is the foundation on which all other systems and processes in an ABA organization stand. Accordingly, managers for quality who can design and implement BIQ control processes that describe, predict and control quality, and sustain through maintaining contingencies at the system and process levels (e.g., Silbaugh, 2022), can win the support of the entire organization for a change initiative to build a robust quality assurance system that takes precedent over profit. Quality managers can describe, predict, and control ASDQ using organizational behavior management (e.g., Daniels & Bailey, 2014) in four steps. Step one is to select a process that impacts ASDQ. In other words, a process that impacts attainment of professional or consumer outcomes, or financial health. Step two is to describe that process as it is actually implemented. Step three is to identify variables predicted to increase cultural practices that positively impact key performance indicators of the process. Step four is to control quality at the process level by experimentally evaluating the effects of interventions on staff performance that produce changes in the value of the key performance indicator until it meets or exceeds the benchmark reliably over time.

Quality Assurance

According to the ASQ website, quality assurance is a part of management focused squarely on instilling confidence in stakeholders that quality requirements of a service or product will be fulfilled (Figure 1.2). In other words, "all the planned and systematic activities implemented within the quality system that can be demonstrated to provide confidence that a product or service will

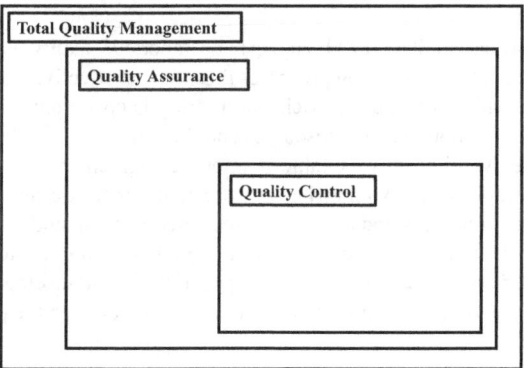

Figure 1.2 The Relationship Between Total Quality Management, Quality Assurance, and Quality Control.

fulfill requirements for quality" (ASQ, n.d.). The father of managing for quality, Joseph M. Juran, defined the prime purpose of quality assurance as, "to serve people who are not directly responsible for conducting operations, but who have a need to know—to be informed as to the state of affairs, and hopefully, to be assured that all is well" (Juran, 1995, p. 627).

For clinical staff of ABA autism service organizations, that means assurance that the organization's culture will provide them with everything they need to implement effective behavioral interventions. For consumers that means assurance that their expectations for improvements in quality of life will be met or exceeded by the service. For third-party payors such as insurance companies, that means assurance that their expectations for the value of care provided to beneficiaries by the service provider will be met.

Quality assurance systems in human service settings are comprised of three basic elements: standards, monitoring, and response mechanisms (Bradley & Bersani, 1990).

Standards

In developing standards, Bradley (1990) recommends adhering to four criteria: consistency, flexibility, clarity, and measurability. The consistency criterion is met if standards can be applied fairly and equitably across programs. The flexibility criterion is met if the standard allows enough flexibility to support innovation and respond to individual needs. The clarity criterion is met if the standard contents are easily communicated. The measurability criterion is met if the standard can be monitored with standardized measurement.

Monitoring

For monitoring, Bradley (1990) suggests designers of quality assurance systems must develop monitoring processes that are cost effective, reliable, valid, timely, and which include feedback. Monitoring is cost effective if it can be implemented without wasting resources and the utility of the data justifies the expenditure. Monitoring is reliable if interrater agreement can be obtained at an acceptable level. Monitoring is valid if the measure used to monitor compliance with the standard reflects the phenomenon under observation. Monitoring is timely if it is captured fast enough and soon enough to enable an immediate response. Feedback is appropriate in monitoring if there are built-in means for getting information about performance to the provider.

Response Mechanisms

Bradley (1990) explained that response mechanisms should be reasonable, credible, and constructive, offer certainty, and demonstrate utility. Response mechanisms are reasonable if the problem and the response to the problem are proportional. These mechanisms are credible if the service provider views the people generating responses to quality assurance data as credible. Response mechanisms are constructive if responses to monitoring data result in improvements in quality. Response mechanisms offer certainty to the extent that responses from the quality assurance system are swift and certain if a provider puts the wellbeing of consumers at risk. Response mechanisms have utility to the extent that quality assurance information generated through monitoring is accessible to and can be addressed through planning and policy development.

Avoiding Problems

In the design of such a system, Bradley (1990) explained that many problems can be avoided in the design of quality assurance systems in human services' settings by focusing on the following objectives:

. . . assure that providers of human services have the capability to provide an acceptable level of service; . . . assure that client services are provided consistent with accepted beliefs about what constitutes good practice; . . . assure that a commitment of resources produces a reasonable level of service from the point of view of the consumer as well as the one supplying the funds; . . . assure that the services that are provided have the intended effect; . . . assure that the legal and human rights of people with disabilities are protected.

(p. 8)

The Quality Trilogy

Quality assurance is achieved by managing for quality. On May 20, 1986, Joseph M. Juran identified a manufacturing quality crisis, and laid out his view of a "universal approach to managing for quality" called the "quality trilogy". The quality trilogy had a major influence on the field of quality. The three components of the trilogy are quality planning, quality control and quality improvement.

Quality Planning

Juran explained that quality planning is "the process for preparing to meet quality goals" and the end result of quality planning is "a process capable of meeting quality goals under operating conditions" (Juran, 1986, p. 3). Additionally, quality planning is, "effectively the design stage during which an organization establishes an understanding of its target customer's needs, defines the features and specifications of the product or service, and devises the processes that will deliver on those needs" (DeFeo, 2019).

Quality Control

This is "the process for meeting quality goals during operations" and the end result of the process is "conduct of operations in accordance with the quality plan" (Juran, 1986, p. 3). Additionally, quality control involves "periodic checks and inspections, and tracking metrics to ensure the process is in control and meeting specifications. Where defects are identified, root causes need to be identified to enable corrective and preventative action" (DeFeo, 2019). The website for the ASQ defined quality control as, "part of quality management focused on fulfilling quality requirements" (ASQ, n.d.). And, "While quality assurance relates to how a process is performed or how a product is made, quality control is more the inspection aspect of quality management. In other words, "the operational techniques and activities used to fulfill requirements for quality" (ASQ, n.d.).

Quality Improvement

This is "the process for breaking through to unprecedented levels of performance", the end result of which is "conduct of operations at levels of quality distinctly superior to planned performance" (Juran, 1986, p. 4). Additionally, "While organizations may expect to achieve incremental improvements by day-to-day means, breakthrough quality improvement involves the identification of areas where processes can be optimized, and the organized creation of beneficial change in order to attain measurably improved performance" (DeFeo, 2019).

Summary

Simply put (Figure 1.3), quality planning involves designing processes and setting standards, quality control consists of reducing variability and improving performance until the quality plan is met, and quality improvement consists of taking actions to increase quality beyond expectations.

Managing for Quality in ABA Autism Service Delivery

Managing for quality in an ABA autism service organization can be conceptualized by analogy to the quality trilogy. Quality planning is the process for preparing to deliver ABA services that meet standards. The end result is a process capable of meeting standards when ABA services are delivered. Quality control is the process for meeting quality goals during ABA service delivery.

Quality Trilogy

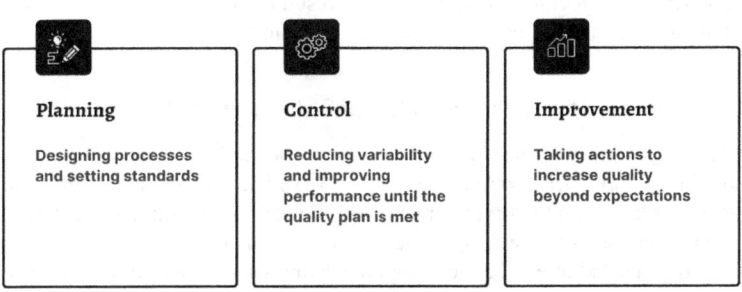

Planning

Designing processes and setting standards

Control

Reducing variability and improving performance until the quality plan is met

Improvement

Taking actions to increase quality beyond expectations

Figure 1.3 Quality Planning, Control, and Improvement in the Quality Trilogy.

MANAGING FOR QUALITY IN ABA

Quality Planning

Process: The process for preparing to deliver ABA services that meet standards.
End Result: A process capable of meeting standards when ABA services are delivered.

Quality Control

Process: The process for meeting quality goals during ABA service delivery.
End Result: Delivery of ABA services that meet standards.

Quality Improvement

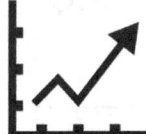

Process: The process for breaking through to unprecedented levels of clinical quality.
End Result: Conduct of ABA service delivery in a manner that far exceeds quality standards.

Figure 1.4 Managing for Quality in ABA Service Delivery.

The end result is the delivery of ABA services that meet standards. Alternatively, quality improvement is the process for breaking through to unprecedented levels of clinical quality. The end result is the conduct of ABA service delivery in a manner that far exceeds quality standards.

Behavioral Intervention Quality and the Quality Trilogy

Behavioral interventions are manipulations of environmental variables to produce desired behavior change. Research explicitly addressing quality control over behavioral interventions in ABA autism service settings was largely nonexistent as of this writing. A definition of behavioral intervention quality (BIQ) is needed to ensure the search for definitions of BIQ does not prevent scientific progress on this topic and the development of methods for controlling BIQ. Accordingly, the following definition shown in Figure 1.4 is offered as a starting point, to be debated and refined and perhaps even replaced in future research: A behavioral intervention is high-quality to the extent that practitioners consistently demonstrate high procedural fidelity and high interobserver agreement over repeated observations of focused behavioral intervention. In other words, independent variable quality plus dependent variable quality over time equals BIQ.

Procedural Fidelity

Procedural fidelity is an indicator of independent variable integrity and a measure of independent variable quality (St. Peter et al., 2023). It is the extent to which

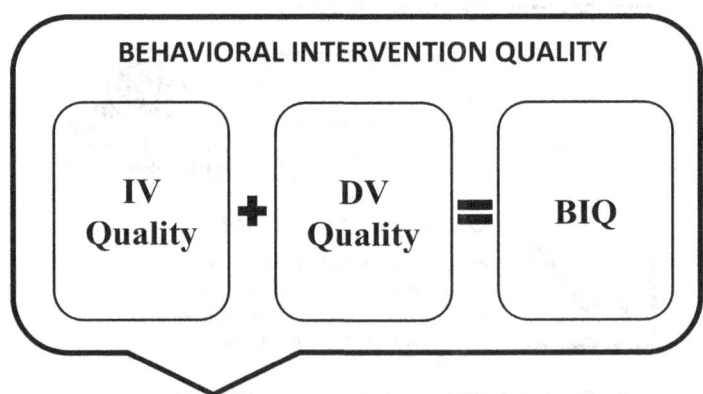

Figure 1.5 Behavioral Intervention Quality Is Independent Variable Quality Plus Dependent Variable Quality.

a behavioral intervention is implemented as planned (e.g., Cooper et al., 2020). In the context of the current quality control model, procedural fidelity indicates the extent to which the quality plan for a behavioral intervention is met. For example, implementing a behavioral intervention with 70% accuracy is low procedural fidelity, 71–89% accuracy is moderate, and 90% accuracy is high. Procedural fidelity assessments contribute to believability that behavioral data were collected under the condition specified by the behavioral intervention protocol. Methods of procedural fidelity assessment derive from three general types: self-report, permanent product measurement, and direct observation (e.g., Sanetti & Kratochwill, 2009). Direct observation is the most flexible, adaptable, direct, comprehensive, and defensible method for assessing procedural fidelity, making it ideally suited for high-stakes evaluations (e.g., Sanetti & Kratochwill, 2009).

Interobserver Agreement

Interobserver agreement is an indicator of dependent variable integrity and behavior measurement quality (Kostewicz et al., 2016). It is the extent to which at least two independent observers collect data on a target response and the data are in agreement (e.g., Cooper et al., 2020). Low-, moderate-, and high-interobserver agreement are indicated with the same value thresholds (i.e., 70%, 71–89%, 90–100%) as with procedural fidelity assessment. In the context of the current quality control model, interobserver agreement is another indicator of the extent to which the quality plan for a behavioral intervention is met. The methods for assessing interobserver agreement vary procedurally and in terms of their methodological rigor. Benefits of assessing interobserver agreement include determining observer competence, detecting observer drift, and ruling out changes in measurement as an explanation for variability in graphed behavior data.

Focused Behavioral Interventions

The current model of quality control pertains to the implementation of focused behavioral interventions (Steinbrenner et al., 2020). Comprehensive treatment models "consist of a set of practices designed to achieve a broad learning or developmental impact on the core features of ASD" (p. 426; Odom et al, 2010a). The Denver model (Rogers et al., 2000) is an example. Procedural fidelity and interobserver agreement assessments however are not applicable to broad sets of practices. These assessments are applicable to determining the independent and dependent variable integrity of focused behavioral interventions. Focused behavioral interventions are, "practices . . . designed to address a single skill or goal of a learner with autism (Odom et al., 2010b). These practices are operationally defined, address specific learner outcomes, and tend to occur over a shorter time period" (p. 11) than comprehensive treatment models. Examples of focused behavioral interventions are nonremoval of the spoon for food refusal, differential reinforcement for tact training, and chaining to teach shoe tying.

Quality planning, control, and improvement of BIQ for focused behavioral interventions too can be viewed by an analogy to the quality trilogy as illustrated in Figure 1.6.

Quality Planning for BIQ

This is the design of a behavioral intervention that can be implemented at or above independent variable and dependent variable quality standards. For example, a written protocol for the implementation of functional communication training to treat attention maintained challenging behavior. The end result is a behavioral intervention capable of meeting standards when direct treatment is implemented.

○ ○ ○ ○

MANAGING BEHAVIORAL INTERVENTION QUALITY

Quality Planning

Process: The design of a behavioral intervention that can be implemented at or above IV and DV quality standards (e.g., FCT)
End Result: A behavioral intervention capable of meeting standards when direct treatment is implemented.

Quality Control

Process: The application of IOA/treatment integrity checks to ensure the behavioral intervention meets IV and DV quality standards during direct treatment (e.g., IOA/integrity of FCT).
End Result: Implementation of a behavioral intervention that meets IV and DV quality standards.

Quality Improvement

Process: Management of cultural contingencies that accelerate rates of DV and IV quality control practices to achieve unprecedented levels of DV and IV quality (e.g., increased incidence of high IV/DV quality).
End Result: Cultural practices in quality control that far exceed quality standards and prior expectations.

○ ○ ○ ○

Figure 1.6 Behavioral Intervention Analog of the Quality Trilogy.

Quality Control of BIQ

This is the application of interobserver agreement and procedural fidelity assessments to ensure that the behavioral intervention meets independent and dependent variable quality standards during direct treatment. For example, interobserver agreement and procedural fidelity assessment of functional communication training. The end result is the implementation of a behavioral intervention that meets independent and dependent variable quality standards. In other words, functional communication training consistently implemented with 90% procedural fidelity and interobserver agreement.

Quality Improvement of BIQ

This is the management of cultural contingencies (e.g., metacontingencies; Glenn et al., 2016) which increase dependent and independent variable quality control practices to achieve unprecedented levels of BIQ. For example, the increased incidence and prevalence (e.g., Biglan, 1995) of high independent and dependent variable quality in an organization's clinical services' department. The end result is persistent cultural practices that far exceed quality standards and continue to occur despite service recipients and employees coming and going over time.

Chapter Summary

ABA autism service providers need practical methods for controlling the quality of their behavioral interventions. Quality is parity between expected and actual outcomes. As a fundamental cultural practice, humans have managed quality for thousands of years. Quality assurance provides confidence to all stakeholders that high-quality services will be delivered. Quality assurance systems in human services such as ABA autism therapy are comprised of standards, monitoring systems, and mechanisms for responding to variability in those systems. Quality assurance is achieved with organization-wide quality management involving planning, control, and improvement. The first step in building a quality assurance system in ABA autism service delivery with an ASDQ framework is establishing a process for exerting quality control over BIQ. High-quality behavioral intervention can be achieved with quality control over procedural fidelity and interobserver agreement.

References

American Society for Quality. (n.d.). *The history of quality.* https://asq. org/quality-resources/history-of-quality.

Baer, D. M., Wolf, M. M., & Risely, T. R. (1968). Some current dimensions of applied behavior analysis. *Journal of Applied Behavior Analysis, 1*, 91–97. https://doi. org/10.1901/jaba.1968.1-91

Biglan, A. (1995). *Changing cultural practices: A contextualist framework for intervention Research.* Context Press.

Bradley, B. J., & Bersani, H. A. (1990). *Quality assurance for individuals with developmental disabilities: It's everybody's business.* Paul H. Brooks Publishing Co.

Cochran, C. (2015). *ISO 9001:2015 in plain English.* Paton Professional.

Cooper, J. O., Heron, T. E., & Heward, W. L. (2020). *Applied behavior analysis* (3rd ed.). Pearson Education.

Daniels, A. C., & Bailey, J. S. (2014). *Performance management: Changing behavior that drives organizational effectiveness* (5th ed.). Aubrey Daniels International.

DeFeo, J. A. (2019, April 15). *The Juran trilogy: Quality planning.* https://www.juran.com/blog/the-juran-trilogy-quality-planning/

Glenn, S., Malott, M., Andery, M. A. P. A., Benvenuti, M., Houmanfar, R., Sandaker, I., Todorov, J. C., Tourinho, E. Z., & Vasconcelos, L. (2016). Toward consistent terminology in a behaviorist approach to cultural analysis. *Behavior & Social Issues, 25,* 11–27. https://doi. org/10.5210/bsi.v25i0.6634.

International Organization for Standardization. (2015). *Quality management principles.* https://www.iso.org/publication/PUB100080.html

International Organization for Standardization. (n.d.). *ISO 9001:2015 quality management systems: Requirements.* https://www.iso.org/standard/62085.html

Juran, J. M. (1986). The quality trilogy: A universal approach to managing for quality. *Quality Progress, 19*(8), 19–24. https://asq.org/quality-progress/articles/the-quality-trilogy?id=fd76da805e434c93837d640f98461e98

Juran, J. M. (1995). *A history of managing for quality: The evolution, trends, and future directions of managing for quality.* ASQC Quality Press.

Juran, J. M. (2019, March 4). *The history of quality.* https://www.juran.com/blog/the-history-of-quality/

Kostewicz, D. R., King, S. A., Datchuk, S. M., Brennan, K. M., & Casey, S. D. (2016). Data collection and measurement assessment in behavioral research: 1958–2013. *Behavior Analysis: Research and Practice, 16*(1), 19–33. http://dx.doi.org/10.1037/bar0000031

Merriam-Webster.com. (2023). Quality. *Merriam-Webster.* Retrieved December 24, 2023, from https://www.merriam-webster.com/dictionary/quality

Morris, C., Conway, A. A., Becraft, J. L., & Ferrucci, B. J. (2022). Toward an understanding of data collection integrity. *Behavior Analysis in Practice, 15,* 1361–1372. https://doi.org/10.1007/s40617-022-00684-x

Morris, C., Jones, S. H., & Oliveira, J. P. (2024). A practitioner's guide to measuring procedural fidelity. Advance online publication. *Behavior Analysis in Practice.* https://doi.org/10.1007/s40617-024-00910-8

Mueller, J. (Host). (2023, April 11). What is quality? With Dr. Bryant Silbaugh (No. 69) [Audio podcast episode]. *Building Better Businesses in ABA.* https://buildingbetterbusinessesinaba.buzzsprout.com/1896922/12631031-episode-69-what-is-quality-with-dr-bryant-silbaugh

Odom, S. L., Boyd, B. A., Hall, L. J., & Hume, K. (2010a). Evaluation of comprehensive treatment models for individuals with autism spectrum disorders. *Journal of Autism and Developmental Disorders, 40*(4), 425–436. https://doi.org/10.1007/s10803-009-0825-1

Odom, S. L., Collet-Klingenberg, L., Rogers, S. J., & Hatton, D. D. (2010b). Evidence-based practices for children and youth with autism spectrum disorders. *Preventing*

School Failure: Alternative Education for Children and Youth, 54(4), 275–282. https://doi.org/10.1080/10459881003785506

Porter, M. E., & Twisberg, E. O. (2006). *Redefining health care: Creating value-based competition on results.* Harvard Business School Press.

Qiupeng, J., Meidong, C., & Wenzhao, L. (1995). Ancient China's history of managing for quality. In J. M. Juran (Ed.), *A history of managing for quality: The evolution, trends, and future directions of managing for quality* (pp. 1–31). ASQC Quality Press.

Rogers, S. J., Hall, T., Osaki, D., Reaven, J., & Herbison, J. (2000). The Denver model: A comprehensive, integrated educational approach to young children with autism and their families. In J. Handleman & S. Harris (Eds.), *Preschool education programs for children with autism* (2nd ed., pp. 215–232). PRO-ED.

Sanetti, L. M. H., & Kratochwill, T. R. (2009). Toward developing a science of treatment integrity: Introduction to the special series. *School Psychology Review, 38,* 445–459. https://www.proquest.com/scholarly-journals/toward-developing-science-treatment-integrity/docview/219656532/se-2

Silbaugh, B. C. (2022). Discussion and conceptual analysis of four group contingencies for behavioral process improvement in an ABA service delivery quality framework. *Behavior Analysis in Practice, 16,* 421–436. https://doi.org/10.1007/s40617-022-00750-4

Silbaugh, B. C. (2024). A crisis and a compass: Towards an industry-wide research agenda on ABA autism service quality. ResearchGate. http://dx.doi.org/10.13140/RG.2.2.11593.76644

Silbaugh, B. C., & El Fattal, R. (2022). Exploring quality in the applied behavior analysis service delivery industry. *Behavior Analysis in Practice, 15,* 571–590. https://doi.org/10.1007/s40617-021-00627-y

Slocum, T. A., Detrich, R., Wilczynski, M., Spencer, T. D., Lewis, T., & Wolfe, K. (2014). The evidence-based practice of applied behavior analysis. *Behavior Analyst, 37,* 41–56. https://doi.org/10.1007/s40614-014-005-2.

Steinbrenner, J. R., Hume, K., Odom, S. L., Morin, K. L., Nowell, S. W., Tomaszewski, B., Szendrey, S., McIntyre, N. S., Yücesoy-Özkan, S., & Savage, M. N. (2020). *Evidence-based practices for children, youth, and young adults with autism.* The University of North Carolina at Chapel Hill, Frank Porter Graham Child Development Institute, National Clearinghouse on Autism Evidence and Practice Review Team.

St. Peter, C. C., Brand, D., Jones, S. H., Wolgemuth, J. R., & Lipien, L. (2023). On a persisting curious double standard in behavior analysis: Behavioral scholars' perspectives on procedural fidelity. *Journal of Applied Behavior Analysis.* https://doi.org/10.1002/jaba.974

Taylor, F. W. (1911). *The principles of scientific management.* Harper & Brothers Publishers.

2   Make a Quality Plan

ABA therapy is the gold standard in the assessment and treatment of individuals with autism because when validated behavioral interventions are high-quality and evidence-based, they work! Quality control over my behavioral interventions is one of the best things I have accomplished in my practice. With quality control, I can trust more that the RBTs on my autism care teams will implement the interventions I design. I am more confident that my interventions can be implemented with the evidence-based practice of ABA (Slocum et al., 2014). When I inspect my clients' graphed behavior data, I am completely comfortable interpreting those data and my ability to make data-based decisions that will result in changes in my clients' behavior in the desired direction. When a skill acquisition target appears ready to master, I do not doubt it and I am comfortable mastering that target and introducing the next. I am happier, more optimistic, and energized to do more for my clients. My RBTs' skills consistently improve over time with repeated practice conducting quality control cycles across multiple exemplars of behavioral interventions. With more confidence in my RBTs' abilities, I can design more innovative and individualized behavioral interventions. With a quality plan for controlling the quality of your behavioral interventions, you can too!

You are officially equipped with foundational quality concepts of management, assurance, planning, control, and improvement. Now you are ready to develop a quality plan for ensuring that controlling BIQ is feasible and sustainable in the context where you work. Your initial quality plan will consist of (1) a quality control protocol, (2) job aides, (3) mastery criteria, and (4) a team. Completion of this chapter constitutes your quality plan for implementing quality control over BIQ. When you start the process, your goal will be to work with your RBT(s) in dyads to implement the quality plan to its specifications at the level specified by a mastery criterion.

DOI: 10.4324/9781003475095-2

The 10-Step Protocol for Quality Control by BCBA

Quality control over BIQ with the current model consists of repeated implementation of quality control cycles over time by a BCBA-RBT dyad. A *quality control cycle* is an instance of the quality control process. Each quality control cycle is implemented according to a 10-step standard operating protocol described as follows, illustrated in Figure 2.1.

Step 1. Initiate a Quality Control Cycle

A quality control cycle begins with a BCBA or RBT initiating the cycle. For example, the RBT asks the BCBA to "conduct a QC check". A cycle ends with documentation of the outcome. When the BCBA-RBT dyad is new to the process, cycles are initiated by the BCBA by asking the RBT to conduct a quality control check. When quality control cycles become routine, RBTs should transition to initiating QC checks.

Example: "After 15 minutes of establishing rapport for the day with the RBT and the client, the BCBA opens their laptop and the RBT asks them to conduct a QC check."

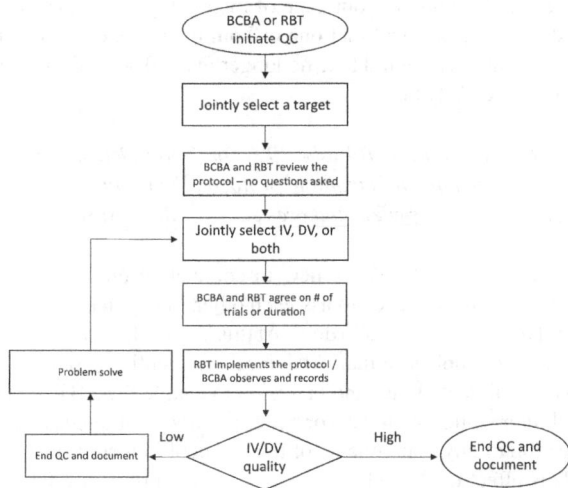

Figure 2.1 Quality Control Cycle Diagram.

Note: BCBA = Board Certified Behavior Analyst; BI = Behavioral Intervention; DV = Dependent Variable; IV = Independent Variable; QC = Quality Control; RBT = Registered Behavior Technician.

Step 2. Select a Target

Also referred to as selecting a protocol. The RBT and BCBA jointly select a skill acquisition target, such as tacting common household items. This step should take no more than 15 seconds to complete for a BCBA-RBT dyad fluent in quality control over BIQ.

Example: "The RBT and BCBA decide to conduct a quality control check on functional communication training targeting tangibly maintained challenging behavior."

Step 3. Protocol Review

The BCBA and RBT independently review the target protocol as written either in an electronic data collection platform such as CentralReach™, Catalyst™, or Motivity™; or on a paper data sheet. When both BCBA and RBT have reviewed the protocol, they explicitly confirm to each other that they have read the protocol and are ready to begin. Verification that BCBA and RBT have just read the protocol helps prevent extraneous variables (i.e., undue influences on the dependent variable that are out of the behavior analyst's control) from influencing the outcome of the quality control cycle, such as a recent update to the protocol that one or both members of the dyad may not have noticed. This step should take no longer than 30 seconds to complete for a fluent BCBA-RBT dyad.

Example: "The RBT and BCBA take 30 seconds to independently review the functional communication training protocol, then explicitly tell each other they completed their review and are ready for the next step."

When BCBA-RBT dyads are new to conducting quality control cycles, they can slip into the tendency to ask each other, "Do you understand the protocol?" or "Do you know what to do?". At this step of the quality control cycle, it is important to emphasize that behavioral intervention protocols should be written with sufficient clarity and precision to enable the RBT to perform the behavioral intervention with 90% or better accuracy without asking questions or clarification of any components of the protocol in a conversation with the BCBA. This effect of the behavioral intervention protocol reflects the technological dimension of ABA (Baer et al., 1968). Put another way, the behavioral intervention should be written such that it functions as a discriminative stimulus with antecedent control over the RBT's performance of the target behavioral intervention. In the presence of the BCBA, feedback confirming procedural fidelity or interobserver agreement at or above your organization's standard (e.g., 90%) was demonstrated by the RBT should function as conditioned positive reinforcement for engaging in quality control cycles (see Figure 2.2). Improvements in the learner's behavior, or improvements in graphed data representing learner behavior change should function as conditioned reinforcement for the RBT performing the behavioral intervention as planned, over time, in the absence of the BCBA. The ideal functional relation between the behavioral intervention protocol, RBT implementation, and learner behavior change or graphed behavior data are illustrated in Figure 2.3.

This of course also hinges on whether the BCBA supervisor writes protocols for behavioral interventions that are effective! But that is a topic for another book. Deviations in procedural fidelity and interobserver agreement

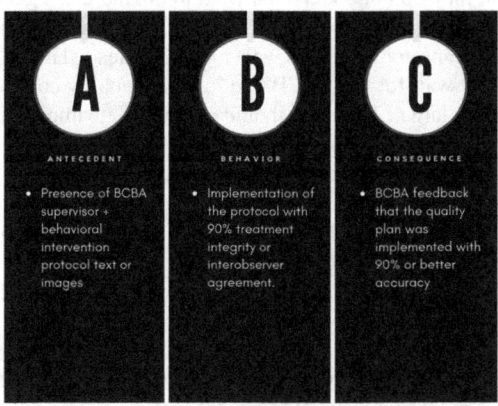

Figure 2.2 The ABCs of RBTs Implementing Behavioral Intervention Protocols With Procedural Fidelity or Interobserver Agreement in the Presence of the BCBA.

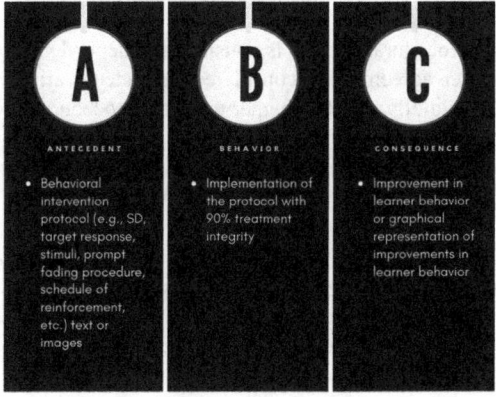

Figure 2.3 The ABCs of RBTs Implementing Behavioral Intervention Protocols With High Procedural Fidelity in the Absence of the BCBA.

evoked by the target protocol should be treated as faulty discriminative stimulus control that can potentially be addressed through edits of the protocol between quality control cycles. If you discuss the protocol with the RBT and then modify the protocol accordingly, make sure you conduct another quality control cycle on the revised target in a subsequent session per the standard quality control cycle so you can verify that modifications to the protocol, not your conversation with the RBT, more effectively exert discriminative stimulus control over their behavioral intervention implementation.

When you and the RBT review the behavioral intervention protocol, if the RBT tells you they do not understand what to do, there is a good chance that they have seen the protocol before you arrived for supervision and they chose not to follow the protocol, and to wait for you instead. That is too late. The RBT should not wait for their BCBA to initiate a quality control cycle to get clarification on a target. The RBT should communicate immediately with you if they encounter a protocol they do not think they can implement. Structuring quality control cycles such that the BCBA-RBT dyad goes straight from reading the protocol, to agreeing on the number of trials and proceeding with behavioral intervention, teaches the RBT to ask for clarification earlier in a different context, quickly show you the behavioral intervention so you can make your observations, and give you rapid access to RBT behavior you can shape. As a result, you can revise the protocol instructions based on what the RBT did after reading it, not what the RBT "said" after they read it. The BCBAs should not write protocols that evoke the RBT's verbal behavior about the protocol during a direct treatment session. They should write protocols that evoke the RBT immediately performing the behavioral intervention.

Step 4. Select Procedural Fidelity, Interobserver Agreement, or Both

In this model, procedural fidelity is considered independent variable quality and interobserver agreement is considered dependent variable quality. The RBT and BCBA jointly decide whether to assess procedural fidelity, interobserver agreement, or both if the team is highly experienced in quality control cycles. This step should take no more than 30 seconds to complete for a fluent BCBA-RBT dyad.

Example: "The RBT and BCBA briefly discuss the data and what it has been like implementing the target since the last supervision session. The BCBA and RBT decide it would be most beneficial at the moment to conduct a quality control check on procedural fidelity."

Step 5. Define the Observation Period

The BCBA and RBT agree on how many trials of the behavioral intervention the RBT will conduct (e.g., ten trials), or for how long the RBT will implement the behavioral intervention (e.g., five minutes). Use the former for discrete operant arrangements and the latter for free-operant arrangements. At least five discrete trials or five minutes of free-operant intervention is recommended to ensure data are collected on an adequate sample of the RBT and learner's behavior. It is often helpful for the BCBA to keep track of time and trials so that the RBT can focus on implementation. This step should take no longer than 15 seconds to complete for a fluent BCBA-RBT dyad.

Example: "The RBT and BCBA decide to assess procedural fidelity for 5 minutes of implementation of functional communication training with a reinforcer duration of 30 seconds."

Step 6. RBT Initiates Implementation

Next the RBT explicitly tells the BCBA that they are starting to implement the behavioral intervention. This step is important because there are a lot of competing stimuli for the BCBA to attend to but they need to watch the RBT continuously during the observation period. It is also important to ensure accurate timing (i.e., tracking the duration of the observation period) and completion of the correct number of trials during the observation period. This step should take no more than 5 seconds to complete for a fluent BCBA-RBT dyad.

Example: "The RBT says 'I'm setting the timer and starting now' and the BCBA acknowledges."

Step 7. Implementation and Observation Period

The RBT implements the behavioral intervention protocol for the predetermined number of trials or minutes, while the BCBA independently observes implementation. If the dyad is assessing procedural fidelity, the BCBA collects data on the RBT's implementation of the behavioral intervention using the estimation method of procedural fidelity assessment described later. If the dyad is assessing interobserver agreement, the BCBA collects trial-by-trial data on the learner's responses independent of the data collected by the RBT and uses a standard calculation to determine interobserver agreement (Cooper et al., 2020). It is highly recommended that RBTs collect trial-by-trial data routinely during quality control cycles to prevent accidentally running too many or too few trials and to run trials at a pace that the BCBA can keep up with.

Example: "The BCBA observes the RBT continuously during the observation period and prepares to collect estimation data on procedural fidelity at the end of the observation."

Step 8. Analysis

The BCBA and the RBT discuss the data (i.e., outcome of interobserver agreement or procedural fidelity assessment) and problem solve if there is a need for improvement in BIQ. This step may include modification of the protocol, modifications to the environment, the provision of materials (e.g., stimuli) that may have been missing during implementation, remediation of RBT performance deficits through additional skill training (i.e., to be completed between successive cycles with cycles serving as opportunities to repeatedly rehearse), or other problem-solving steps depending on the circumstances. This step should typically take no more than 1–2 minutes to complete for a fluent BCBA-RBT dyad.

Example: "The outcome of the procedural fidelity assessment was an estimated 75% correct. The BCBA and RBT note that the protocol described the schedule of reinforcement and prompting strategy, but these components were lacking technological precision. Accordingly, the BCBA agreed to edit those components for clarity before running another cycle of quality control on functional communication training."

Step 9. Documentation and Progress Monitoring

Before moving on to another supervisory responsibility, or initiating another quality control cycle, the BCBA closes the quality cycle by quickly documenting the outcome through a process. If quality control of BIQ is being managed by a clinical director, the BCBA should submit a form to the clinical director for monitoring, analysis, and feedback. However, if the BCBA-RBT dyad conduct quality control cycles independent of a clinical director or other quality manager, the BCBA can document the outcomes in a simple Microsoft Excel® spreadsheet.

Example: "The BCBA submits a quality control check Google Form™ to the organization's Google Drive™ folder where all of the BIQ quality control data are stored".

Take a moment to list the types of information you would want to document in a form after a quality control cycle. Do not design a form that will take a BCBA more than 30 seconds to complete once they are fluent with the process. Examples of obvious data include the name of the BCBA, the name of the RBT, the client's identification code, the type of cycle completed (e.g., IV or DV check), and the outcome (e.g., 70% interobserver agreement).

How might this form affect how consistently the BCBA will document quality control cycles?

How long do you think it will take the BCBA to complete and submit the form, and why?

Step 10: Repeat Cycles to Meet the Benchmark

Improvements in the efficiency of implementing quality control cycles and outcomes of quality control cycles will come with repeated practice by dyads who get along and enjoy working with each other. The dyad should complete multiple back-to-back cycles of quality control on a given target, time permitting, until the designated benchmark for procedural fidelity and interobserver agreement set by the organization, are met. I recommend a benchmark of 90% procedural fidelity and 90% interobserver agreement. In other words, for a given target such as functional communication training described in the example above, BCBA-RBT dyads should conduct more than one quality control cycle in a single supervision session, and continue to conduct cycles until the benchmark is met or they run out of time. Repeated implementation of quality control cycles on a single target by the dyad maximizes the probability that the dyad will contact reinforcement for engaging in quality control in the form of improvements in procedural fidelity, improvements in interobserver agreement, and improvements in client progress.

Example: "The BCBA-RBT dyad's first cycle yields 40% interobserver agreement. The BCBA submits a form to document the outcome of the cycle. Then the dyad discusses revisions in the operational definition of the target response, runs another cycle, and attains 90% interobserver agreement. The BCBA submits a form to document the outcome of the second cycle and moves on to other supervisory responsibilities".

Summary

If implemented as described earlier, the quality control cycle protocol should be very easy to implement by the BCBA-RBT dyad. If it feels rushed, strained, overly complicated, or forced, the dyad is doing something wrong and they should take some time to figure out what the issues are and consider asking a colleague to observe the dyad engaging in this practice. When BCBA-RBT dyads first start using this model to control BIQ, the most important outcome is not high procedural fidelity and interobserver agreement. It is that the dyad enjoys their time together, collaborates well, communicates well, walks away from the experience feeling like they accomplished something important, and that they repeat the process soon thereafter.

Some BCBAs might opt to initially survey their RBTs to assess their perspective on the new model for controlling BIQ. What are some questions you might want to ask your RBTs to determine whether they find the model acceptable and valuable?

The Estimated Procedural Fidelity Assessment

I believe that the success of this model of quality control over BIQ hinges heavily on the use of the estimated procedural fidelity assessment (EPFA) described as follows (see Figure 2.4). To establish a lasting cultural practice such as routine checks of BIQ capable of overcoming all of the competing responsibilities facing a BCBA in clinical supervision sessions, BCBAs need an extremely simple, straightforward, low-effort method for assessing procedural fidelity of any intervention, anywhere, at any time. As such, the EPFA was developed for practical reasons.

In the EPFA, we don't care about the precision of procedural fidelity assessment for outcomes of the assessment less than 70%. If the outcome of a procedural fidelity assessment is estimated at 70%, we don't care if that estimation is off plus or minus 5%, 10%, or 15%. It doesn't matter because anything less than 90% is treated as needing improvement. That is, an esti-mated procedural fidelity score of less than 90% indicates that modifications of some sort are needed, and another quality cycle should be conducted to verify that the modifications improve the quality of the behavioral interven-tion. A procedural fidelity score that is equal to or greater than 90% suggests that no modifications of the target protocol are needed although there is some room for minor improvement. Allowing for a range of estimated pro-cedural fidelity (i.e., 70–100%) in your system for documenting outcomes allows for variability in the data to monitor trends in procedural fidelity values over time.

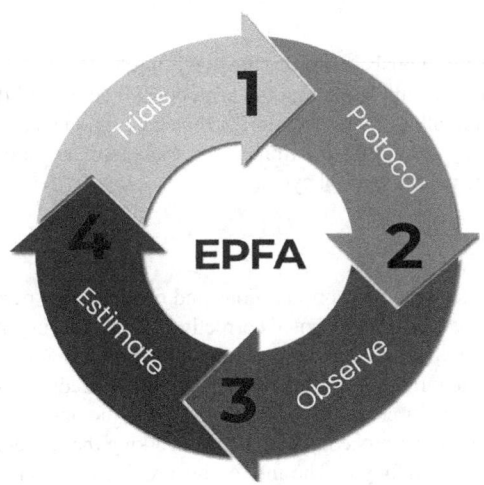

Figure 2.4 Visual Depiction of the EPFA.

The steps of the EPFA are as follows:

Step 1

The BCBA notes the observation type. For example, the RBT will implement trials or implement intervention for a duration of time. Trial-based observations are more appropriate for discrete operant targets such as tacts, matching, joint attention, and receptive instructions. Duration-based observations are more appropriate for free operant targets such as manding, functional communication training, spontaneous tacting, spontaneous eye contact, and play skills taught in naturalistic formats.

Step 2

The BCBA reads the components of the target protocol and notes the number of components. For example, a target protocol that specifies the method, setting, SD(s), target response(s), instructional stimuli, implementer, pacing/timing, reinforcement schedule, prompt fading strategy, and error correction procedure, has specified ten components. By completing many quality control cycles, I learned that by standardizing how behavioral intervention protocols are written, such as standardizing terminology and the number of intervention components, it is possible to reduce variability in procedural fidelity. By setting the number of intervention components at ten, it is also really easy to estimate the percentage procedural fidelity after an observation period without a calculator.

Step 3

The BCBA continuously observes the RBT implement the target protocol until the RBT stops implementing the protocol. I recommend that the BCBA and RBT do not talk to each other during the observation and implementation period as a way to eliminate extraneous variables that could influence the outcome of the quality control cycle.

Step 4

The BCBA reflects on their observations and estimates the percentage of the components that were implemented correctly "overall" during the observation period. For example, if the RBT generally implemented 8/10 of the components during each trial, the BCBA would estimate procedural fidelity at 80%. You can also monitor errors of commission during the observation.

Practice estimating procedural fidelity by working these examples. The first example is completed for you. The answers are provided at the end of the chapter.

Example Protocol:

Step	Description
1. Setting	Living room at home
2. SD	Presence of preferred items
3. Target response	Vocally mand for the preferred item with a recognizable approximation, single-word
4. Reinforcement	Fixed-ratio 1 schedule of positive reinforcement
5. Prompting	Transition from errorless vocal model prompts to partial vocal model prompts to a 10 second time-delay
6. Error correction	None
7. Implementer	RBT
8. Pace	Contrive a mand opportunity every 30 seconds without manding or after 30 seconds of reinforcement for the previous mand

The observation duration: Five minutes of mand training
Observations: The RBT used ~60 second reinforcer durations and implemented the intervention in the kitchen.
Procedural fidelity estimate: 75%

Practice Protocol 1:

Step	Description
1. Setting	Backyard
2. SD	Shown a bucket, shovel, or chair and asked "What is it?"; randomly rotated across trials
3. Target response	Says bucket, shovel, or chair within five seconds of the SD
4. Reinforcement	Fixed-ratio 1 schedule of positive reinforcement thinned to a variable-ratio 2
5. Prompting	Transition from errorless vocal model prompts to partial vocal model prompts to a ten-second time-delay following the presentation of each stimulus.
6. Error correction	None
7. Implementer	RBT
8. Pace	30-second ITI

The observation duration: Ten trials
Observations: The RBT could not find the shovel, they strictly alternated between bucket and chair SDs, and the schedule of reinforcement was FR 2.
Estimate procedural fidelity: _____

Practice Protocol 2:

Step	Description
1. Setting	Clinic room 2
2. SD	"What is your name?" "And your name is?" "Your first name is?" randomly rotated across trials.
3. Target response	Learner independently says their first name.
4. Reinforcement	Fixed-ratio 1 schedule of positive reinforcement thinned to a variable-ratio 2
5. Prompting	Transition from errorless vocal model prompts to partial vocal model prompts to a two-second time-delay following the presentation of each stimulus. After three consecutive correct responses to time-delay trials, discontinue all prompts.
6. Error correction	Organization standard EC
7. Implementer	RBT
8. Pace	30-second ITI, accelerated to five-second intertrial intervals interspersed with a variety of mastered intraverbal targets as prompts are faded.

The observation duration: Ten trials

Observations: The RBT used the EC incorrectly on two trials, prompts were not errorless for roughly half of the trials and the learner is unable to respond independently; the RBT only used the SD "What is your name?" for the current target, but did a good job of interspersing mastered intraverbal targets across trials.

Estimate procedural fidelity: _____

Practice Protocol 3:

Step	Description
1. Setting	Clinic room 2 bathroom
2. SD	Told "Wash your hands"
3. Target response	Learner independently performs the last step of the handwashing chain as defined in the task analysis—dry hands on towel
4. Reinforcement	Fixed-ratio 1 schedule of positive reinforcement using the preferred tangible from a multiple stimulus without a replacement preference assessment
5. Prompting	Backward chaining
6. Error correction	None
7. Implementer	RBT
8. Pace	Separate back-to-back contrived trials by one minute

The observation duration: Five trials

Observations: The RBT ran the target in clinic room 3 bathroom.

Estimate procedural fidelity: _____

Make Job Aides

Job aides are antecedent stimuli that can be designed to increase the likelihood an employee will perform a job skill as expected. When a BCBA-RBT dyad is new to conducting quality control checks of BIQ, a job aide can be useful for both the BCBA and the RBT. The purpose of this particular job aide is to help ensure that the BCBA-RBT dyad precisely completes every step of a quality control cycle correctly and in the right order. A job aide can take many different forms. I recommend creating a job aide for the steps of the quality control cycle by printing a single page, one-sided, laminated, list of the steps, and providing a copy to each of the dyad members. Remember to gradually fade out the job aide so that the dyad can perform quality control cycles independently, correctly, and efficiently. Figure 2.5 is a sample job aide you can use now.

You can develop your own job aide by jotting down your ideas below.

_____

_____

_____

_____

_____

_____

_____

_____

QUALITY CONTROL CYCLE
Checklist

- BCBA or RBT initiate QC
- Jointly select a protocol
- BCBA and RBT review the protocol
- Jointly select IV, DV, or both
- BCBA and RBT agree on # of trials conducted or duration
- RBT implements the protocol for # trials and BCBA observes and records
- If IV/DV quality is high, end QC and document result
- If IV/DV quality is low, end QC and document result, then problem solve and repeat cycles until IV/DV quality is high

Figure 2.5 Quality Control Checklist.

For many RBTs, implementation of quality control cycles might be the first time they have come into contact with the following terms:

* Independent variable
* Dependent variable
* Procedural fidelity
* Interobserver agreement

If you refine the terminology in the target protocols to be more conceptually systematic and technological before you implement quality control cycles, it is likely you will be introducing additional terms that many RBTs are not familiar with. It is unfortunate, but you will meet many RBTs in your career who have either never heard terms such as "motivating operation", "schedule of reinforcement" and "time-delay" in the field or who have worked in settings where the use of these terms was not reinforced. It will be very difficult to implement the evidence-based practice of ABA in your behavioral interventions and attain high interobserver agreement and procedural fidelity with quality control cycles if you do not use technical behavior analytic terms in your protocols. I highly recommend making a vocabulary list for your RBTs containing key terms and their definitions, and providing these materials as job aides the day you introduce your RBTs to the current model (i.e., your quality plan).

Consider taking a moment here to list some of the terms you think your RBTs may need job aides for. In each column, write the term in the box on the left, and the definition of the term in the box on the right. I wrote the first one for you! Remember, you are writing this for RBTs.

Dependent variable	An aspect of behavior you measure to assess behavior change over time. (e.g., correct/incorrect, duration, count)

Prepare to Manage Embarrassed RBTS

When you conduct quality control cycles for the first time, you may discover that your RBT does not know what they are doing. And they might feel embarrassed—as if they have been doing their job incorrectly all along. More specifically, you may discover that the protocols for your behavioral interventions do not exert as much antecedent stimulus control over the RBT's performance as you hoped for. That is okay. This discovery is an opportunity to dramatically improve the RBT's work life, their career, and your client's clinical outcomes. Accordingly, it's important to prepare for how you are going to help your RBTs cope with the explicit identification of gaps in their ability to run behavioral interventions as written, make it safe to make mistakes, and get them the resources, knowledge, and training they need to remediate their performance deficits and start obtaining high procedural fidelity and interobserver agreement scores. Take a moment to jot down some notes about how you might do this. Do not think of it as set in stone. This exercise is intended only as a nudge to get you thinking about what you might do. How are you going to send the message that "We're all in this together"?

_____

_____

_____

_____

_____

_____

_____

_____

Date	Cycle	Client Code	RBT Initials	IV Integrity Estimate	IOA
10-01-2023	1	JaDe	TH	90	
10-02-2023	2	JaDe	TH		85
10-03-2023	3	FrEu	RD		100
10-04-2023	4	NaBo	FE	65	
	5	NaBo	FE	85	
	6	NaBo	FE	90	
10-05-2023	7	JaDe	TH	95	

Figure 2.6 Example of an Excel® Sheet a BCBA Supervisor Can Use to Monitor the Outcomes of Quality Control Cycles Over Time.

Note: Each date represents a different supervision session. Multiple quality control cycles were completed in some sessions (e.g., 10/4/2023). Each row represents a different quality control cycle. For dates with multiple rows, multiple cycles were completed on that date during the same supervision session. It may be helpful to calculate and monitor the monthly average outcome value as well. There are also other ways to organize the data. The BCBA supervisors should also graph the data to enable data-based decisions about implementation of quality control cycles. IOA = interobserver agreement.

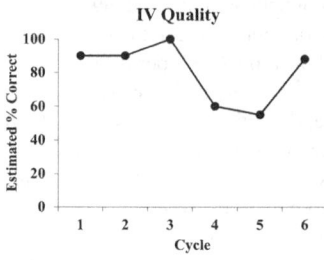
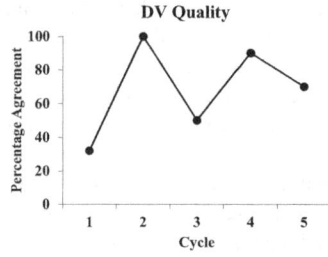

Figure 2.7 Sample Equal Interval Line Graphs for Monitoring Outcomes of Quality Control Cycles Over Time.

Note: DV = dependent variable integrity or the outcome of an interobserver agreement assessment. IV = independent variable integrity or the outcome of a procedural fidelity assessment. This sample represents how to display quality control cycles over time combining all RBTs and learners in the chronological order in which they were conducted.

Documentation

You need a system for documenting the outcomes of quality control cycles to serve two purposes in your practice. You need to record and aggregate quality control cycle data for making decisions about how to improve the quality of your behavioral interventions. You also need those data for monitoring quality of BIQ over time. A simple electronic spreadsheet will do. I used Microsoft Excel™ when I first started piloting the current model. I recommend structuring your spreadsheet as illustrated in Figure 2.6. Sample equal interval line graphs for graphically displaying the data are illustrated in Figure 2.7. It may be helpful to graph quality control data separately for individual RBTs and for individual learners.

Mastery Criteria

Mastery criteria are important for determining when the dyad has mastered the clinical practice of routinely implementing BIQ quality control cycles. I recommend a mastery criterion of five consecutive quality control checks completed by the BCBA-RBT dyad across at least two clients, in two contexts, in the absence of any job aides. Note that attainment of this quality plan means repeated accurate implementation of quality control cycles targeting BIQ, not necessarily the demonstration of high BIQ. High BIQ is attained when quality control cycles result in the implementation of behavioral interventions (e.g., quality plans for teaching mands, tacts, play skills, self-care skills) with high procedural fidelity and high interobserver agreement. In other words, in accordance with plans for BIQ.

The Team

The minimal team for implementing quality control over BIQ is a BCBA-RBT dyad. No other team members are necessary. In some cases, it may be helpful to solicit support from a clinical director, but it is not necessary. To scale implementation of quality control over BIQ in an organization requires at least one clinical director (i.e., manager for quality), and that is discussed in further detail later in a subsequent chapter.

Now that you know what control over BIQ requires, take some time to list a couple of RBTs on your caseload. For each RBT, list reasons you think they might be a good candidate for collaborating with you on piloting this model of quality control. Then list some reasons they might not be a good candidate. After completing this exercise, choose the RBT candidate who is likely to be most supportive of your efforts and whom you think has the skills needed to help you make the model work. For example, an RBT who is full-time, enrolled in a master's program in behavior analysis, and has three years of experience, may be a better candidate than a part-time RBT with three months of experience and who is not quite sure ABA is the career path for them. If you need more space to write, pull up a word document or some scratch paper and jot your thoughts down there.

RBT Name:_____

Why they might be the best candidate:

_____

_____

_____

Why they might NOT be the best candidate:

_____

_____

_____

RBT Name:_____
Why they might be the best candidate:

_____

_____

_____

Why they might NOT be the best candidate:

_____

_____

_____

Prepare to Lead

Before you approach the best RBT candidate to collaborate on piloting this new process, take some time to write a persuasive, compelling, and supportive description of how you will motivate your RBT to collaborate. If you will use behavioral skills training (BST) to teach your RBT how to conduct quality control cycles, think of this exercise as writing the rationale and information you will present to the RBT before modeling aspects of the process.

Forget the idea of "buy in" or trying to get the RBT to "understand" what you want them to do. Approach this exercise as a radical behaviorist. You need an establishing operation in place for your RBT that will momentarily increase the likelihood they will challenge themselves and try something new, and increase the value of reinforcers you expect them to contact as a result of implementing quality control cycles. Help your RBT imagine the benefits of learning to control the quality of their behavioral interventions and client clinical outcomes beyond the data.

Roofers do not merely lay down shingles. Roofers keep homeowners safe and protect their investment by providing them with a roof that can withstand extreme weather and prevent damage to the interior of their home. The RBTs do not merely implement behavior interventions to change behavior and generate data. They implement behavioral interventions with high procedural fidelity and interobserver agreement over time to progressively improve the quality of their learner's life. Consider telling your RBT that you will only make protocol modifications to targets going forward after, in collaboration with you, they have demonstrated high procedural fidelity and interobserver agreement. Then follow through on that promise!

_____

_____

_____

_____

_____

_____

Give careful thought to how you will teach your RBT to experience corrective feedback as positively reinforcing for participating in the conversation, and arrange a discriminative stimulus and establishing operation for completing the next quality control cycle. In the author's experience, it takes very little convincing of RBTs to continue conducting quality control cycles after trying it out a couple times. That is because as a result of completing multiple quality control cycles and experiencing improvements in procedural fidelity and interobserver agreements, those outcomes are likely to function as reinforcement for the behavior of both dyad members. When you make your first target protocol modification following high procedural fidelity and interobserver agreement, make sure you draw your RBT's attention to that consequence for their behavior.

Now take a moment to describe how you might give corrective and supportive feedback to the RBT at the end of each quality control cycle that yields substandard performance (i.e., low procedural fidelity or interobserver agreement). Think about how you will make it okay for the RBT to make mistakes, how you will shape their performance in a manner they appreciate, and how you will make sure they feel valued as a result of participating in the process.

_____

_____

_____

_____

_____

_____

Chapter Summary

Quality control over BIQ begins with a quality plan for BCBA-RBT dyads conducting quality control cycles in routine practice. The quality plan is comprised of ten steps: initiate a quality control cycle, select a target, review the protocol, select independent or dependent variable integrity to assess, define the observation period, RBT-initiated implementation of the protocol, an implementation observation period, analysis of the outcome, documentation, and repeated cycles within a supervision session until benchmark procedural fidelity and interobserver agreement scores are attained. This plan utilizes a four-step estimation method of procedural fidelity assessment to work around common barriers to assessing procedural fidelity routinely. Job aides can help the BCBA-RBT dyad master the implementation of quality control cycles. The BCBAs should set up for success by identifying the right RBT(s) to start piloting the process with and giving some initial consideration to the contingencies the BCBA will need to put into place to reinforce RBT participation. The BCBA may need to take some initial steps to manage RBT embarrassment if quality control cycles initially reveal substandard performance. Documentation of quality control cycles is essential for progress monitoring outcomes of quality control cycles and making adjustments to maximize procedural fidelity and interobserver agreement over time.

Answers to EPFA Practice Questions

1. 75
2. 60
3. 88

References

Cooper, J. O., Heron, T. E., & Heward, W. L. (2020). *Applied behavior analysis* (3rd ed.). Pearson Education.
Slocum, T. A., Detrich, R., Wilczynski, M., Spencer, T. D., Lewis, T., & Wolfe, K. (2014). The evidence-based practice of applied behavior analysis. *The Behavior Analyst, 37,* 41–56. https://doi.org/10.1007/s40614-014-005-2.

3 Quality Control by BCBA

Congratulations, you have a plan for controlling BIQ with methods that really work! Now it is time to implement quality control to achieve the quality plan in practice! This chapter will guide you through logistics, the first few days of implementing quality control of BIQ, leveraging your data to motivate your RBTs to improve BIQ, sharing your data with a clinical director, and inspiring others to follow your lead.

Logistics

Quality control cycles are conducted during sessions in which a BCBA supervises an RBT implementing behavioral interventions during direct treatment with a client. This can be accomplished in-person or remotely using a videoconferencing application such as Zoom® or Google Meet®. In most cases, it will be easier to pilot the current model in-person. More experienced BCBA-RBT dyads will have success remotely as they maintain the cultural practice of controlling BIQ.

Selecting a Target

If you are a BCBA, at this stage of your career you have probably walked into a supervision session, observed your RBT attempt to implement a target, and noticed that your RBT seems completely lost! You spent all that time and hard work writing the behavioral intervention protocols in your practice-management system but what your RBT is implementing looks nothing like what you programmed. Don't panic, it happens to all of us! The BCBA-RBT dyads will quickly realize that quality control checks with the current model don't seem to make sense when implementation of a skill acquisition or behavior-reduction target is way off from the actual behavioral intervention protocol. For example, when the protocol for the behavioral intervention is grossly incomplete or the RBT has almost completely misinterpreted the protocol. In

DOI: 10.4324/9781003475095-3

those instances, don't waste time completing an entire quality control cycle. First, remediate any major deficiencies in the behavior intervention protocol and RBT repertoire, then initiate a quality control cycle.

Behavioral Interventions Are Quality Plans

Your ten-step plan for conducting quality control cycles is a quality plan for the practice of controlling BIQ. In contrast, a quality plan for BIQ is the design of a behavioral intervention that can be implemented at or above independent variable and dependent variable quality standards. When you write out the components of a behavioral intervention (e.g., SDs, target responses, schedule of reinforcement) you are writing a quality plan for skill acquisition. The quality plan must be written such that it is sufficiently precise, complete, and clear that a trained RBT can reasonably be expected to implement the plan with few questions or committing few errors (i.e., the technological dimension of ABA; Baer et al., 1968).

Quality control of BIQ is the application of interobserver agreement and procedural fidelity assessments to ensure that the behavioral intervention meets independent and dependent variable quality standards during direct treatment. For example, independent and dependent variable quality of functional communication training. In other words, quality control of BIQ is engaging in practices that ensure the quality plan for the skill acquisition or behavior reduction target is demonstrated by the RBT during the observation portion of the quality control cycle. High-quality behavior intervention is equivalent to accurate implementation of the quality plan. The effectiveness of the intervention, such as whether it produces the desired skill acquisition or behavior reduction, is not BIQ. Rather, the effectiveness of an intervention is dependent on BIQ. High BIQ is necessary for behavioral interventions to produce their desired effects.

Quality improvement of BIQ is the management of cultural contingencies (e.g., metacontingencies; Glenn et al., 2016) which increase dependent- and independent variable quality control practices to achieve unprecedented levels of BIQ such as the increased incidence and prevalence of high independent and dependent-variable quality throughout an organization's clinical services' department. The end result is cultural practices that far exceed quality standards. Because behavioral intervention plan implementation cannot exceed 100% accuracy, quality improvement does not apply to BIQ at the performer level. Quality improvement occurs at the group or organizational level and is indicated by exceeding a quality plan for the incidence or prevalence of quality control checks and BIQ levels attained by a group or organization over time. This idea is discussed in greater detail in the chapter on managing quality control by manager or director.

Leading and Shaping RBT Performance

Every quality control cycle is an opportunity to bring your RBT's clinical decision making into contact with the positive reinforcement produced by improvements in learner behavior. Don't waste the opportunity a quality control cycle provides by sweating the small stuff, giving too much corrective feedback, or blaming your teammate for substandard quality. Frame every quality control cycle as an opportunity for the BCBA-RBT dyad to bond, to collaborate, to help each other, and to provide high-quality behavioral intervention. Every deviation from the components of a behavioral intervention discovered during a quality control cycle is a gift—a wonderful opportunity to work with your colleague to deliver something better in the next cycle. BCBAs have more power, privilege, and responsibility than RBTs. Recognize that fact about your role as a BCBA and take responsibility for as much of the error or deviations in quality you can. Your RBT will appreciate you, trust you, follow your lead, and do everything they can to deliver high procedural fidelity and interobserver agreement.

The Journey: From Day 1, to Mastery, to Becoming an Influencer in Your Organization

Day 1

To hit the ground running on day 1, spend some time reviewing the quality plan the night before. Make sure you have your job aide(s) and progress monitoring data sheet ready to go. Make sure you have largely memorized what you are going to say to the RBT to motivate their involvement. With any luck, you will motivate them right out of the gate. "Do you mind if we try something new? I think you'll like it!" are magical words. That might be all you need to get your RBT going with the first couple of quality control cycles! If you are a full-time BCBA, you will probably supervise more than one RBT that day. If you are piloting with two RBTs, try to conduct a quality control cycle at least once with each RBT. If things go really well, try for two quality control cycles!

The first time you attempt to complete a quality control cycle, choose a behavioral intervention that is easy for your RBT to implement correctly, and take it nice and slow. In the quality plan above, I have suggested how long each step should take to complete, or the expected duration of the step is implied. For example, you observe the RBT implement the behavioral intervention for five minutes. If you are piloting quality control cycles for the first time, don't expect to complete each step as quickly as suggested. It might take you 15–20 minutes to complete the first cycle, especially if your RBT has questions. Allocate as much time as you can to answering the RBT's questions, and make sure the conversation ends on a high note. Lead with gratitude and compliment the RBT on their collaboration and their willingness to be flexible and try new things in service of their client and their organization's culture.

Days 2–3

On days 2–3, you should start becoming more comfortable with completing steps of the quality control cycle in order, and so should your RBTs. Make it a point to complete at least one cycle per supervision session. You will also discover some of the kinks in the methods you use to collect data on quality control checks. That is good because this is the time to refine your methods. At the end of each day, consider calling your RBTs, checking in on them, and asking them what they thought about conducting quality control cycles with you now that they have had time to think about this new process. Ask open-ended questions to learn anything you can do differently or better to help them enjoy the process and master their steps of the process.

Weeks 1–3

Here are some indicators over the next three weeks that things are probably going well:

(1) You should have refined your quality control check data collection methods and found a graphical data display that clearly illustrates (a) the rate at which you have conducted quality control cycles and (b) the effects of those cycles on target procedural fidelity and interobserver agreement.

(2) You should have your RBTs' full support. For example, they fully cooperate with conducting quality control cycles, you get no complaints, and they seem to be enjoying the process.

(3) You should have clear evidence that quality control cycles are associated with large improvements in procedural fidelity and interobserver agreement on multiple targets with all the RBTs who have been involved in the process.

(4) You should begin to see reductions in variability in the data paths for at least some of the behavioral interventions for which you have achieved high procedural fidelity and high interobserver agreement.

(5) You should have met mastery criteria. That is, you should have met the quality plan in practice, with all of the RBTs you have involved in the process.

Months 2–3

If you have managed to routinely complete quality control cycles for three or more weeks across more than one RBT and client, and met mastery criteria for quality control cycles, congratulations, this is an extraordinary accomplishment! You have overcome many barriers and introduced a new clinical cultural practice to your organization with the power to inspire an increase in your organization's investment in quality assurance.

If you are a clinical supervisor, I recommend continuing to control BIQ with the current model for 2–3 months before formally presenting your quality data with the clinical director. Make sure you balance your quality control efforts across behavioral interventions within clients, across clients, and across RBTs so that quality control over BIQ is balanced across the contexts in which you work. If you are a clinical director piloting the model with your RBTs, do the same before formally presenting your data and the process with the BCBA clinical supervisors who report to you. The larger the data set, and the more consistent, sustained, and effective practice you can demonstrate to your colleagues, the easier it will be to convince them to follow your lead by adopting quality control over BIQ in their own clinical practice. Try to complete roughly 25 dependent-variable quality control checks and 45 independent variable quality control checks before presenting your data to your colleagues. Chances are, your colleagues have already heard what you have been up to and will be interested to learn more!

Influence

Depending on your standing in your ABA organization, you may be in a position to leverage your BIQ data to inspire your colleagues, clinical director, or both, to follow your lead and try to replicate what you have accomplished. Here are some tips:

Maintain Really Nice Graphs of Your Data

Make sure your data are well organized and your graphs follow best practices in graphical display. Turn to your textbooks and the scientific literature for guidance on best practices in displaying data graphically, and follow those guidelines closely. Jon Bailey and Mary Burch offer some very straightforward recommendations in their second edition text on research methods in ABA (Bailey & Burch, 2018). If your graphs look great, there is a better chance that your colleagues will take your data seriously.

Make a Very Brief PowerPoint™ Presentation of the Current BIQ Model

Have the presentation ready to go at a moment's notice. Never pass an opportunity to share what you have accomplished with your colleagues. Invest in high-quality images, keep the text brief, and focus your presentation on

(a) the model, (b) the data, and (c) benefits of quality control over BIQ. Present case examples of behavioral interventions you improved with quality control cycles and the benefits to the client. Bailey and Burch's text will help with this too.

Say "YES!" to Anyone Who Asks for Training

If a colleague asks to observe you implementing quality control cycles, or asks you to train them, agree immediately and do anything you can to support their success. Including sending them the link to purchase this book!

Meet With Your Clinical Director

Ask your clinical director if they have time to meet with you for a brief presentation on your current quality control cycle data. In your request, specify the length of the presentation, the main points, what the clinical director will gain from participating in the meeting, and a list of all the days and times you are available to meet with them that or the following week. Tell them you are willing to work around their schedule. If you are successful at securing a meeting with your clinical director, practice your presentation as many times as you can, with colleagues or friends willing to critique and give you candid feedback on your performance, until you can fluently deliver the presentation without notes. You might only get one chance, so come prepared to be both persuasive and influential! Bailey and Burch's first edition of "25 Essential Skills & Strategies for the Professional Behavior Analyst" (2010) is a great resource for expert tips on giving persuasive and influential presentations. At the end of your presentation, emphasize how easy it is to begin conducting quality control cycles on BIQ and list 2–3 next steps you propose taking in collaboration with the clinical director to teach quality control over BIQ to other BCBA supervisors in the organization. With any luck, the clinical director will ask you to train them! If that happens, you have struck gold!

Chapter Summary

With the quality plan from Chapter 2 in place, you are ready to start implementing quality control cycles over BIQ. You can do this remotely or in-person, but the latter is a highly recommended initial modality. Major RBT performance deficiencies should be remediated before conducting quality control cycles. Behavioral intervention protocols are themselves individual quality plans. The quality plan for a behavioral intervention is met when quality control cycles demonstrate that the plan is implemented with high procedural fidelity and interobserver agreement over time. Quality improvement of BIQ occurs at the group or organizational level. Quality control cycles should be viewed by BCBA-RBT dyads as valuable opportunities to bond, collaborate, and help each other provide high-quality behavioral interventions. Days 1–3 of conducting quality control cycles are about getting comfortable with the process, learning to implement the steps of quality control cycles in order, and refining your progress monitoring methods. Weeks 1–3 are about mastering correct implementation of quality control cycles. Months 2–3 are about continuing to progress monitor quality control cycle frequency and outcomes, achieving high procedural fidelity and interobserver agreement, and organizing and preparing to leverage those data to inspire your colleagues to follow your lead.

References

Baer, D. M., Wolf, M. M., & Risley, T. R. (1968). Some current dimensions of applied behavior analysis. *Journal of Applied Behavior Analysis, 1*, 91–97. https://doi. org/10.1901/jaba.1968.1-91

Bailey, J., & Burch, M. (2010). *25 essential skills & strategies for the professional behavior analyst: Expert tips for maximizing consulting effectiveness.* Routledge.

Bailey, J. S., & Burch, M. R. (2018). *Research methods in applied behavior analysis* (2nd. ed). Routledge.

Glenn, S., Malott, M., Andery, M. A. P. A., Benvenuti, M., Houmanfar, R., Sandaker, I., Todorov, J. C., Tourinho, E. Z., & Vasconcelos, L. (2016). Toward consistent terminology in a behaviorist approach to cultural analysis. *Behavior & Social Issues, 25*, 11–27. https://doi. org/10.5210/bsi.v25i0.6634

4 Managing for Quality

Clinical directors manage and supervise the services that clinical BCBAs and RBTs provide. In the current model, clinical directors are also managers for quality (i.e., quality managers). They describe, predict, and control the quality of behavioral interventions implemented by BCBA-RBT dyads. Quality managers should look for BCBA-RBT dyads engaging in cultural practices that positively impact service quality, and reinforce those practices. Quality managers indirectly achieve control over BIQ through their unique position by differentially reinforcing the clinical cultural practices of BCBA-RBT dyads that positively impact ASDQ, such as engaging in quality control cycles to increase procedural fidelity and interobserver agreement for their behavioral interventions.

BIQ Quality-Management Process

The BIQ quality management process is illustrated in Figure 4.1.

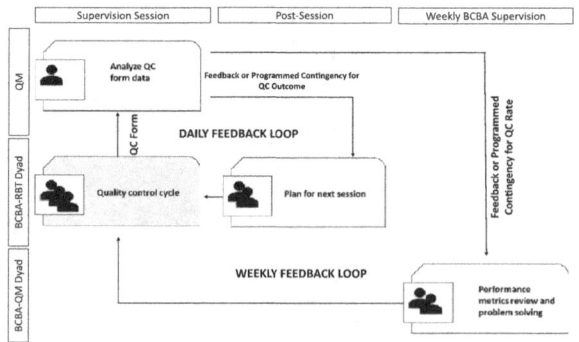

Figure 4.1 Prototypical Process Map of the BIQ Quality Management Process.
Note: QC = quality control; QM = quality manager.

DOI: 10.4324/9781003475095-4

Quality management of BIQ begins with an instance of a quality control cycle during a direct treatment session conducted by the BCBA-RBT. As shown in a prototypical example of this process in Figure 4.1, at the end of the quality control cycle, the BCBA documents the outcome and submits a form to the quality manager. The quality manager analyzes the data, sends feedback electronically to the BCBA-RBT dyad to close the daily feedback loop, and the BCBA, RBT, or both, make plans for improving quality in the next session. In this sample process map, the BCBA supervisor and quality manager meet weekly to review quality metrics. The quality metrics are data collected on key performance indicators within an organization's ASDQ framework which the BCBA has an impact on.

For example, in the current model that could be the last week's rate of QC cycles completed by the BCBA. It is important that the quality manager individualize their practices to the BCBA supervisor. For some, BCBA-QM dyads weekly will work well. For others, bi-weekly or monthly may be appropriate. Some BCBA supervisors may prefer to receive written or graphically depicted feedback rather than verbal feedback in-person.

At New Beginnings Academy, we used Google Forms® for this process. The BCBA submitted a Google Form®, a copy was automatically emailed to the BCBA, and the BCBA forwarded the email from their inbox to the quality manager. On the same day, the quality manager reviewed the contents of the form and replied to the BCBA or both the BCBA and RBT, depending on the outcome of the quality control cycle.

A Standard, a Key Performance Indicator, and a Benchmark

What exactly is the BCBA-RBT dyad expected to do? How often? How well? How will you know when the quality plan for engaging in quality control cycles is met? How will you maintain the cultural practice over time? These important questions can be answered with a standard, a key performance indicator, and a benchmark.

Standard

To demonstrate high-quality ASDQ, organizations need to consistently meet or exceed professional and consumer standards for products, services, and outcomes over time, and maximize financial health. In an ASDQ framework, a standard is, "an official rule, unit of measurement, or way of operating that is used in a particular area of manufacturing or services" (Cambridge Dictionary, n.d.). Standards in an ASDQ framework describe what should be done, but not how well it should be done.

A recommended standard for beginning to manage BIQ quality is: "BCBAs conduct routine quality control cycles on behavioral intervention quality for

PROFESSIONAL STANDARDS

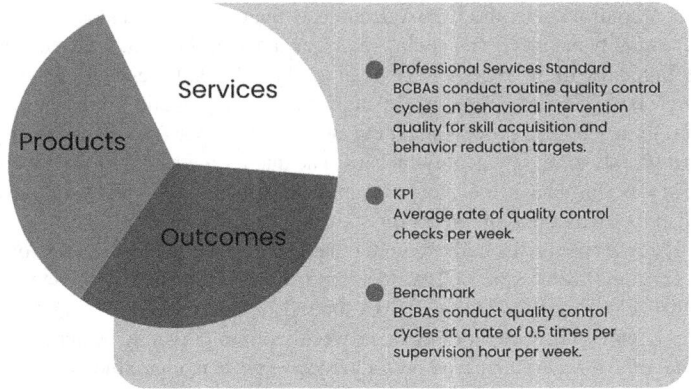

Figure 4.2 Professional Standard for Services, Products, and Outcomes in an ASDQ Framework.

Note: This professional services standard, KPI, and benchmark can be used to promote BIQ in an ASDQ framework.

skill acquisition and behavior reduction targets" (see Figure 4.2). Routine can be operationally defined by the organization in terms of a benchmark, and measured in terms of one or more key performance indicators or "KPIs".

Key Performance Indicator

Parmenter (2015) described four general types of indicators that organizations can track and act on to align employee behavior with critical success factors and the organization's strategic objectives: performance indicators, key performance indicators, result indicators, and key result indicators. This discussion is limited to key performance indicators.

Key performance indicators help management teams determine how employees and processes are performing in relation to critical success factors and strategic objectives, and inform steps they can take to produce significant improvements (Parmenter, 2015). In an ASDQ framework, key performance indicators are useful for daily, weekly, or monthly decision making and performance management needed to attain standards and benchmarks. Broadly used in organizations, key performance indicators are nonfinancial, measured frequently, focus on a specific activity, often reported to the CEO or senior management team, and responsibility is held by a specific team or teams.

The recommended key performance indicator in the current model of managing for quality is the rate of quality control cycles (used interchangeably with the term "quality checks") per week averaged across BCBAs. Equipped with those data, the quality manager can graph the key performance indicator over time and compare the value to the benchmark. When the value of the key performance indicator meets the benchmark, the quality plan has been met at that timepoint and it is time to celebrate! However, remember that quality is dynamic, and the quality plan might not be met the following week if contingencies are not arranged to maintain the cultural practices specified by the plan, competing contingencies are introduced into the environment (e.g., new target introduced), or the intervention does not produce reinforcing client behavior change for the RBT.

Benchmark

The Agency for Healthcare Research and Quality defines benchmark within the context of quality improvement as "performance that is known to be achievable because someone has achieved it" (Agency for Healthcare Research and Quality, n.d.). Within the context of the current model, a benchmark is a value specifying how well or how often a cultural practice should be performed. The main advantage of setting a benchmark for a standard is it enables an organization to establish a reinforcing contingency that maintains performance at or above the benchmark. The recommended benchmark for a clinical services department is "BCBAs conduct quality control cycles at an average rate of 0.5 times per supervision hour per week" for in-home ABA autism service delivery. Center-based ABA autism service providers should more easily meet this benchmark due to having more control over the environment and fewer barriers to engaging in quality control practices.

When outcomes of quality control cycles are consistently below the benchmark for quality levels (e.g., below 90% IOA or procedural fidelity) or the rate of cycles falls below the benchmark for the average rate of quality control cycles per week, this poses an opportunity to further investigate the variables influencing the rate or outcomes of the BCBA-RBT dyad's quality control cycles. Quality managers can use performer level assessment (e.g., McGee & Crowley-Koch, 2021) to identify antecedent and consequence influences on the performance of individual BCBAs or RBTs. They can also use group contingencies to increase the likelihood of achieving the benchmark (Silbaugh, 2023) with process mapping and process improvement (e.g., Luke et al., 2024).

Dashboards and Dashboard Review

The BCBAs need to consistently engage in quality control cycles on a weekly basis to achieve and maintain their quality plans for behavioral intervention. However, competing contingencies and a wide range of barriers occur during supervision sessions that prevent the BCBA from doing this. Accordingly, to maintain BCBAs' quality control practices, quality managers should aggregate BCBA data on quality control (i.e., key performance indicators) and present the BCBA feedback in the form of a quality indicators dashboard (i.e., this can be a simple Excel® spreadsheet) during regularly scheduled 1:1 BCBA supervision meetings. A quality manager's dashboard may contain data on any number of quality indicators, but data on the rate of quality control cycles per supervision hour should be one of them. Per the standard suggested earlier in this book, quality managers should aim to ensure that BCBA supervisors maintain quality control cycles at a rate of 0.5 times per supervision hour. Quality managers can shape BCBA performance gradually by setting stepwise achievable goals and reinforcing goal attainment accordingly.

For example, consider initially setting the target rate at 0.15 time per supervision hour. When the BCBA supervisor meets that goal, increase the target rate to 0.25 times per supervision hour, and ultimately to 0.5 times per supervision hour. Alternatively, the quality manager can collect baseline data on the BCBA's rate of submitting quality control cycle forms, then set goals for shaping higher rates. During the supervision meeting, the BCBA and the quality manager should examine the rate of quality control cycles completed by the BCBA that week, discuss any barriers to meeting the benchmark, and collaborate on plans to maintain or increase the rate of quality control cycles next week.

What to Document

As indicated in the process map of the BIQ quality control process, a procedure for documenting and analyzing quality is needed so that the quality manager can give the BCBA-RBT dyad timely and effective feedback during dashboard review. Managers for quality can create an internal form (e.g., Google Forms) that the BCBA completes at the end of each quality control cycle and submits to the quality manager (i.e., which could be a clinical director). How you design the form will influence the extent to which your BCBA-RBT dyads complete the form consistently. How you design the form also plays a critical role in the quality manager's ability to control quality of BIQ because the data BCBAs enter into the form are the basis for the quality manager's decision making. The quality manager can only act on the data they receive.

For example, a changing criterion design, with the rate of weekly quality control form submissions as the dependent variable, could be useful for experimentally evaluating the quality manager's control over BIQ practices.

Accordingly, recommended features of the form include:

1. Descriptions of the relevant clinical standard and benchmark
2. A description of the process of documenting BIQ by the BCBA

3. Contact information for an administrator who can assist with completing and submitting the form as needed

And entry fields for:

1. BCBA name
2. RBT name
3. Client code (i.e., identifier)
4. The skill acquisition target
5. The type of quality control cycle (i.e., independent or dependent variable)
6. The estimated percentage correct (independent variable quality) or the calculated percent agreement (dependent variable quality)
7. Feedback to the RBT
8. Modifications to the protocol
9. Barriers to achieving 90% agreement or integrity

Validation

Establishing a process for controlling BIQ is no guarantee that quality control cycles will yield accurate procedural fidelity and interobserver agreement data over time. It is possible to establish high incidence, rate, and prevalence of quality control cycles targeting BIQ, without corresponding increases in procedural fidelity and interobserver agreement. Quality managers should validate their model by establishing a benchmark for interrater agreement on quality control cycle outcomes between BCBAs, and engaging in a process of routinely assessing interrater agreement. The recommended benchmark for interrater agreement is: 90% agreement on a mix of independent and dependent variable quality for at least five consecutive supervision sessions, across at least two clients, and at least four targets.

Quality managers can assess interrater reliability and achieve the benchmark for quality control outcomes with the following four step process that can be implemented in-person or remotely via a videoconference application such as Google Meet®.

Step 1. Schedule an Overlap Session

Coordinate a routine overlapping supervision session with the BCBA supervisor. If your overlap will be remote, then you do not have a commute, so you might just schedule the overlap for long enough to conduct a quality control cycle. Ask the BCBA supervisor if they would be comfortable with you assessing interrater reliability. If they express that they are not comfortable at that time and place, ask them for alternative sessions and times in which they would be comfortable until you are able to arrange an overlap session.

Step 2. Complete a Quality Control Cycle

Observe your BCBA-RBT dyad until they begin to conduct a quality control cycle. Ask if you can assess interrater reliability. If they decline, something is wrong and it is beyond the scope of this book! When they agree, perform all of the same steps with the BCBA-RBT dyad (i.e., become a triad!) but collect your data independent of the BCBA.

Step 3. Calculate Interrater Agreement

For procedural fidelity, the quality manager should observe the RBT implement the behavioral intervention. For interobserver agreement, the quality manager should collect those data independent of the BCBA while observing the RBT. Then they should estimate the percentage procedural fidelity or interobserver agreement, independent of the BCBA. Then the they should compare their data to the BCBA's data and use this simple formula to calculate interrater reliability between the quality manager and the BCBA supervisor for either procedural fidelity or interobserver agreement: (smaller % estimate/larger % estimate) * 100.

Step 4. Repeat and Provide Feedback as Needed

Repeat this process until the quality manager and the BCBA meet the benchmark for interrater agreement on quality control outcomes. The quality manager should give feedback between quality control cycles to the BCBA, the RBT, or both, to improve interrater agreement. Once the BCBA-QM dyad (or perhaps one BCBA fluent in quality control cycles and one BCBA in-training) meets the benchmark for interrater agreement on quality control cycle outcomes, the quality manager can consider the BCBA competent to continue routinely assessing procedural fidelity and interobserver agreement on any skill acquisition targets with any client at any time. Teams of BCBA supervisors and quality managers may need to continue to assess interrater agreement on a regular schedule for maintenance.

Controlling Cultural Practices With Quality Management

The hard work of a BCBA-RBT dyad trying to control the quality of their behavioral interventions is a cultural practice to the extent that those behaviors occur with relatively high incidence in the organization over time. To the extent that feedback from the quality manager to the BCBA-RBT dyad controls the future probability of quality control cycles and high BIQ, the relationship between that feedback and those cultural practices is a metacontingency.

Metacontingency

Most BCBAs today have been trained to see the world through a radical behaviorist lens (Johnston, 2014; Skinner, 1974) and interpret human behavior primarily in terms of the operant four-term contingency (i.e., MO-S-R-S). A major focus of any graduate or undergraduate behavior analysis course sequence is for students to learn a molecular approach to the study of functional relations between behavior and environment. For example, I took an introductory course to behavior analysis online early in my career with the Florida Institute of Technology. In that course, Jose Martinez-Diaz taught me the following approach. First, the behavior analyst identifies the behaver. Then they identify the operant behavior of interest. Then they identify relevant environmental events, and classify those events as antecedents or consequences. Then they repeatedly measure the behavior over time as antecedents and/or consequences are systematically manipulated to evaluate their effects on the behavior using single-subject design methodology.

An advantage of analyzing human behavior in terms of the operant is the ability to solve socially significant problems with the behavior of individual people in the service of those people, their families, the community, and society at large (Cooper et al., 2020). A disadvantage is that the behavior analyst may become myopic in their understanding of human behavior (i.e., overly focused on the analysis of behavior of the individual), fail to recognize variables that influence human behavior at the cultural level (i.e., group, process, system), and attempt to implement behavior change procedures and assessments without consideration of the systems and processes within which interventions are implemented. Quality managers must extend their analysis to the group, process, and systems levels to effectively manage for quality and the concept of the metacontingency can help.

In the ASDQ framework and the current model of quality control, it will be useful to define a system as a "network of connecting processes that work together to accomplish the aim of the system" (Furterer & Wood, 2021, p. 266), and a behavioral system as one in which the principal components of its subsystems, processes, subprocesses, and so forth are employees working together to accomplish the aim(s) of the behavioral system (Malott & Garcia, 1987).The ABA autism service organizations are systems of operational, clinical, financial, and other behavioral subsystems working together to deliver ABA services. The behavior of employees and their coordination determine in-part how well the system achieves its service goals. In other words, their cultural practices. Process is defined here as "a series of interrelated actions taken to transform a concept, a request, or an order into a delivered product or service" and, "an activity or group of activities that takes an input, adds value to it, and provides an output to an internal or external customer" (Furterer & Wood, 2021, p. 366).

Within the clinical behavioral subsystem of ABA service delivery, the management of clinical quality control cycles represents a process which converts BIQ plans into the cultural practice of engaging in high-quality behavioral interventions. Thinking in behavior analytic terms about the systems and processes in which behavior occurs can help BCBA supervisors conduct quality control cycles in a manner that is well received by processes that depend on the outcome of clinical supervision (i.e., quality management), and can help quality managers design systems and processes conducive to description, prediction, and control over the quality of their clinical team's interventions.

The metacontingency is an analog of the operant contingency conceptualized by Sigrid Glenn. The most prominent view of the metacontingency is a two-term contingency as illustrated in Figure 4.3. Metacontingency has recently been defined as, "A contingent relation between (1) recurring interlocking behavioral contingencies having an aggregate product and (2) selecting environmental events or conditions" (Glenn et al., 2016). A metacontingency can be arranged to differentially select for cultural practices in a manner that increases the future probability of desirable cultural practices and decreases the future probability of undesirable cultural practices, and their aggregate products.

The first term in the two-term metacontingency is the culturant (Hunter, 2012). Culturant is a term referring to the dependency between interlocking behavioral contingencies and an aggregate product. Interlocking behavioral

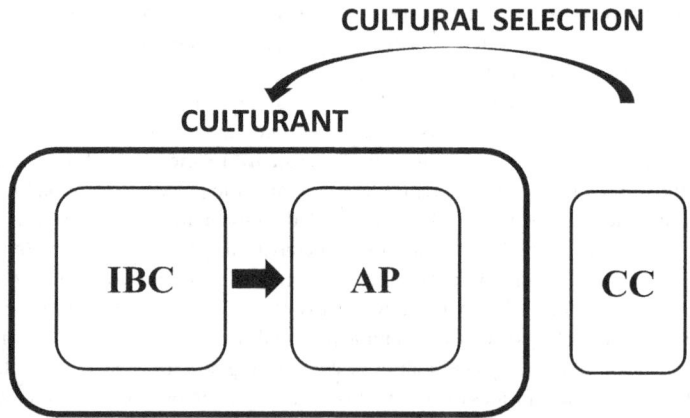

Figure 4.3 Diagram of the 2-Term Metacontingency.

Note: AP = aggregate product; CC = cultural consequence; IBC = interlocking behavioral contingencies.

contingencies are functionally interdependent behaviors exhibited by two or more individuals (i.e., a group) engaging in coordination. Functionally interdependent refers to the fact that each individual engages in behavior or produces results of their behavior that function as controlling antecedents and consequences for the behavior(s) of the other individuals in the group. Interlocking behavioral contingencies produce an aggregate product that cannot be produced by any single member of the group alone. The aggregate product is used by a selector in the context where the culturant occurs to determine when to deliver a cultural consequence. That is, cultural consequences are consequences delivered to all members of the group contingent on one or more characteristics of the aggregate product.

Cultural Selection of Quality Control Cycle Practices

The behaviors of BCBA-RBT dyads providing behavioral intervention can be conceptualized as constituting interlocking behavioral contingencies. In the typical supervision (i.e., protocol modification) session, a BCBA supervisor arrives on site, greets the RBT, they have a conversation, they talk about plans for what will be accomplished in the supervision session, and they coordinate their behavior throughout the session in ways that influence client behavior and result in a record of behavior data and perhaps other permanent products. Those data and other permanent products are the aggregate products of the interaction between the BCBA and the RBT throughout the session. If the BCBA and RBT implement a quality control cycle during the session, a quality control cycle cannot be completed without the BCBA and RBT engaging in behaviors that serve as controlling antecedents and consequences for each other's behavior. The result of a quality control cycle is a completed form containing the percentage procedural fidelity or percentage interobserver agreement resulting from the quality control cycle, in addition to any other information the dyad decides to note.

The form cannot be completed in the absence of the occurrence of the interlocking behavioral contingencies. The production of a completed form is dependent on the dyad engaging in a quality control cycle. Therefore, the quality form is an aggregate product of the quality control cycle and the relation between the interlocking behavioral contingencies (i.e., BCBA initiates a quality control cycle, the RBT and BCBA select a target, they review the protocol) and the aggregate product (e.g., form containing an interobserver agreement score) is a culturant. The aggregate product is submitted to the quality manager by the BCBA supervisor. Aggregate product characteristics can vary over time. For example, procedural fidelity and interobserver agreement data can meet, exceed, or fall short of the benchmark set by the quality manager.

Accordingly, the quality manager has the opportunity to differentially select variations in interlocking behavioral contingencies and their aggregate products (i.e., characteristics of the data such as the procedural fidelity score) remotely by delivering different feedback to the BCBA-RBT dyad contingent on the data (Figure 4.4). When feedback is delivered to the BCBA-RBT dyad (i.e., the daily feedback illustrated in Figure 4.1) contingent on the aggregate product, it can function as a cultural consequence which exerts control over the future probability that the BCBA-RBT dyad will conduct a quality control cycle that produces APs with characteristics that meet or exceed the benchmark.

When feedback is delivered to the BCBA in a meeting with the quality manager, it has the power to influence the rate of quality control cycles completed over time. However, it is important to note that this effect is mediated through the BCBA and that the RBT does not receive feedback on the rate at which the BCBA conducts quality control cycles. In other words, this latter feedback process (i.e., the "weekly feedback loop" illustrated in Figure 4.1) does not constitute a metacontingency. It constitutes an operant contingency between feedback and results (i.e., permanent product) transmitted from BCBA supervisor to quality manager.

There is no guarantee that managing for BIQ will be effective. Managers may need to conduct experimental evaluations of variables that control BIQ for individual BCBA-RBT dyads to determine the conditions under which dyads can consistently meet corresponding benchmarks. Unfortunately, as of the writing of this book I know of no published peer-reviewed studies of the variables that sustain BCBA-RBT engagement in quality control over BIQ in real-world ABA autism service settings. This is an area of research that is completely lacking in the field of ABA and is desperately needed to help ABA autism service organizations build quality assurance systems that deliver high-quality services. ABA autism service organizations must not wait for research to emerge. Even if such studies emerge in the literature, a research-to-practice gap will occur and managers for quality and leaders in ABA autism service organizations will still need to adapt methods validated in the literature and then validate their own models of quality control over BIQ in practice until they discover what works.

Independent Variables

Differences in the contingencies controlled by quality managers now become important to highlight. Feedback to a member of a culturant, such as the BCBA supervisor, feedback to other members of the culturant, such as the RBT, and feedback to the BCBA-RBT dyad (i.e., all members of the culturant), represent different contingencies. They are different independent variables the quality manager can manipulate over time to get the desired results. Other independent variables that may contribute to variability in quality control over BIQ, and which are accessible to the quality manager, include

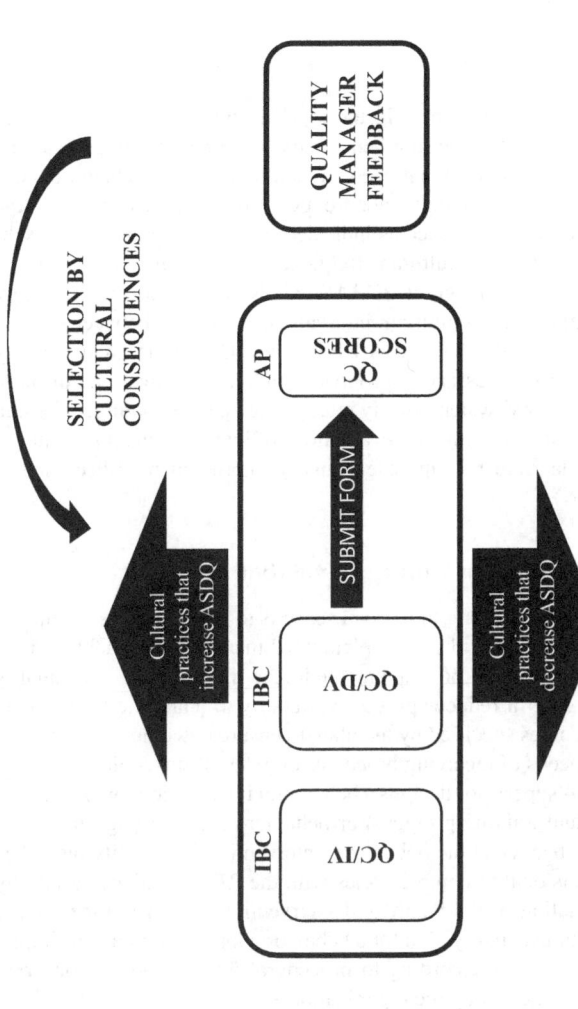

Figure 4.4 Quality Management of Quality Control Cycles.

Note: Quality control cycles are cultural practices consisting of interlocking behavioral contingencies that produce the aggregate product of a quality control form containing the data collected in a quality control cycle. Feedback from the quality manager can differentially select cultural practices that increase quality and decrease cultural practices that decrease quality.

culturant feedback modality (i.e., in-person verbal, print, electronic), the time between AP production and culturant feedback (i.e., feedback delay), and other variables discussed in Chapter 6. These independent variables, and their combination, are likely to produce different effects on one or more relevant culturant dependent variables.

Dependent Variables

Examples of dependent variables in an experimental analysis of variables managers can manipulate to ensure benchmark attainment include behaviors (i.e., employee performances) that occur within interlocking behavioral contingencies, characteristics of aggregate products, culturant incidence (i.e., the frequency of culturant occurrence as indicated by quality control forms submitted), culturant rate (i.e., culturant frequency per unit of time), culturant prevalence (i.e., the percentage of BCBA-RBT dyads who engage in quality control over BIQ) and inter-culturant intervals (i.e., the time between successive culturants produced by a BCBA-RBT dyad). Over time, many quality managers may find it necessary to progress monitor more than one of these dependent variables and systematically manipulate operant contingencies and metacontingencies in experimental evaluations of interventions for maintaining the quality plan and perhaps even quality improvements (discussed in more detail below).

Quality Improvement as Cultural Evolution

To engage in quality planning in a broad sense is to design processes and set standards so that when the plan is implemented there is a reasonable expectation that the process can be implemented according to plan with quality control. Quality control reduces process variability to attain the quality plan and produce outcomes specified by the plan, to ensure outcomes of those processes meet the needs of receiving processes or external stakeholders.

When a BCBA supervisor designs a behavioral intervention for skill acquisition (e.g., a mand training program) or behavior reduction (e.g., treatment for self-injurious behavior) the behavioral intervention is a quality plan. The BCBA implements quality control cycles with the RBT to reduce variability in the implementation of the behavioral intervention and ensure the quality plan is met. Meeting a quality plan for a behavioral intervention means implementing the intervention according to procedural fidelity and interobserver agreement benchmarks set by the organization.

For example, an organization may set a standard that all BCBA-RBT dyads routinely assess procedural fidelity and interobserver agreement during supervision sessions, and a benchmark of 80% procedural fidelity and interobserver agreement on quality control cycle outcomes. Based on this standard and benchmark, quality plans are met when the BCBA-RBT dyad demonstrate 80% procedural fidelity and interobserver agreement on behavioral interventions. They may even demonstrate 90%, or 100%! But these increases in BIQ do not constitute "quality improvement". Quality improvement is an increase in quality beyond expectations. It is expected that many quality control cycles will yield 90% or 100%, even if the organization's benchmark is set lower. Thus, quality improvement cannot be demonstrated at the behavioral intervention level.

Quality improvement is demonstrated at the group or cultural level. Behavior is anything an organism does, and culture is anything a group does. Organizational cultures can be characterized by quantifying incidence and prevalence of cultural practices (Biglan, 1995). *Incidence* is a measure of how often the behavior occurs within a group. If the BCBAs in an ABA autism service organization give a total of five gift cards to their RBTs in one week to recognize those RBTs' accomplishments, the incidence of gift card giving that week is 5. Prevalence is a measure of the proportion of people in the group who engage in the behavior. If there are ten BCBAs, and each of five BCBAs give out one gift card that week, the prevalence of gift card giving was 50% (i.e., five of the ten BCBAs).

Measures of incidence and prevalence can be used to differentiate organizational cultures and subcultures. If one ABA autism service organization greets their families on the first day of therapy with a goodie bag, but other local competitors do not, then the incidence and prevalence of the goodie bag practice differentiates that organization's culture from the competitors. It should become abundantly clear now that the introduction of quality control over BIQ is a variation in cultural practices which represents the evolution of an organization's clinical culture, and that the incidence and prevalence of engaging in quality control over behavioral intervention is a cultural practice that can differentiate one organization's culture from another.

Consider two ABA autism service organizations: organization A and organization B. All of organization A's BCBAs collaborate with occupational therapists in-house in a co-treatment model, and no BCBAs at organization B collaborate with occupational therapists. The incidence and prevalence of collaboration with occupational therapists are high in organization A and absent in organization B. Collaboration with occupational therapists is a cultural practice which defines the clinical culture in organization A due to its relatively high incidence and prevalence in the organization. The rejection of collaboration with occupational therapists is one cultural practice which defines organization B's culture due to its relatively high incidence and prevalence.

Subcultures exist within organizations too. Consider an ABA autism service organization with three clinic sites in a service region: sites 1, 2, and 3. At site 1, 30% of BCBAs use functional analysis to develop function-based interventions for challenging behavior. At site 2, 60% of BCBAs engage in this practice. At site 3, 100% of BCBAs engage in this practice. These values represent the prevalence of this clinical practice. The prevalence of this practice differentiates the clinical cultures across sites. The practice is a prominent feature of the clinical culture at site 3, and an emerging practice at site 1. Or so it seems! Imagine that despite the differences in prevalence, the incidence of functional analysis in the first quarter of the year was 10 at site 3, but 15 at site 2 and 25 and site 1! Although the prevalence of functional analysis is higher at site 3, the incidence is higher at site 1. These too represent differences in the cultural practice between sites. Functional analysis of challenging behavior is a relatively low incidence but highly prevalence practice at site 3 and a relatively high incidence but low prevalence practice at site 1. The most defining features of an organization's culture are high incidence, high prevalence cultural practices that endure with consistency over time.

Quality improvement of BIQ is represented by increases in quantitative measures of cultural practices, such as the incidence or prevalence of quality control cycles and quality control cycle outcomes, relative to a baseline. For example, it is expected that BCBA-RBT dyads can consistently meet quality plans for behavioral interventions by demonstrating 90% or better procedural fidelity and interobserver agreement. An ABA autism service organization could train all of their BCBAs to routinely conduct quality control cycles on BIQ, manage for quality, and achieve and maintain 100% prevalence of this practice over time. However, imagine that three consecutive quarters of quality management indicate a monthly average of 0.15 quality control cycles per supervision hour. If that organization is able to implement a change initiative that produces an increase to 0.5 quality control cycles per supervision hour— a rate of quality control cycles that far exceeds what the organization would otherwise expect in the fourth quarter based on prior data—the increased rate of quality control cycles represents quality improvement of BIQ.

Chapter Summary

Clinical directors can promote quality assurance in an ABA autism service organization by managing for the quality of behavioral interventions with description, prediction, and control of quality control cycles implemented by BCBA-RBT dyads. Managing for BIQ is an ongoing process. In this process, feedback loops enable the manager to leverage operant and cultural selection to reinforce cultural practices that control and ultimately improve BIQ. The clinical director as quality manager references a standard and a benchmark, collects data on BIQ provided by BCBA-RBT dyads, and compares the data to relevant benchmarks. To the extent that differential selection of quality control cycle outcomes is controlled by the quality manager's feedback to BCBA-RBT dyads, control over BIQ by the quality manager constitutes a metacontingency.

Metacontingency control is the cultural selection of clinical cultural practices that contribute positively to quality assurance. The process for documenting quality control cycle outcomes is designed carefully to ensure quality managers receive the information they need to differentially select aggregate products of cultural practices that lead to high-quality behavioral interventions. Quality managers should consider multiple independent and dependent variables in the systematic evaluation of their interventions to ensure their efforts to manage BIQ are successful. Quality managers should regularly assess interrater reliability with BCBA-RBT dyads to ensure quality control cycles are implemented accurately over time and that the data received are valid. To validate the quality control process, quality managers schedule an overlapping supervision session, complete a quality control cycle with the BCBA-RBT dyad, calculate interrater agreement, and repeat as necessary.

Managing for BIQ represents a variant in the evolution of an organization's culture and provides an example of how leaders in ABA autism service organizations can cultivate the cultural practices needed for quality assurance by systematically and empirically occasioning and reinforcing cultural practices as indicated by group-level dependent variables such as incidence and prevalence.

References

Agency for Healthcare Research and Quality. (n.d.). *Comparing scores to a benchmark.* https://www.ahrq.gov/talkingquality/translate/compare/choose/benchmark.html

Biglan, A. (1995). *Changing cultural practices: A contextualist framework for intervention research.* Context Press.

Cambridge Dictionary. (n.d.). *Standard.* https://dictionary.cambridge.org/us/dictionary/english/standard

Cooper, J. O., Heron, T. E., & Heward, W. L. (2020). *Applied behavior analysis* (3rd ed.). Pearson Education.

Furterer, S. L., & Wood, D. C. (2021). *The ASQ certified manager of quality organizational excellence handbook* (5th ed.). ASQExcellence.

Glenn, S., Malott, M., Andery, M. A. P. A., Benvenuti, M., Houmanfar, R., Sandaker, I., Todorov, J. C., Tourinho, E. Z., & Vasconcelos, L. (2016). Toward consistent terminology in a behaviorist approach to cultural analysis. *Behavior & Social Issues, 25,* 11–27. https://doi. org/10.5210/bsi.v25i0.6634

Hunter, C. S. (2012). Analyzing behavioral and cultural selection contingencies. *Revista Latinoamericana de Psicologia, 44*(1), 43–54.

Johnston, J. M. (2014). *Radial behaviorism for ABA practitioners.* Sloan Publishing.

Luke, M. M., Dams, P., & Lichtenberger, S. N. (2024). Improving human-service organizations through process mapping: A tutorial for practitioners. *Behavior Analysis in Practice.* https://doi.org/10.1007/s40617-024-00906-4

Malott, R. W., & Garcia, M. E. (1987). A goal-directed model for the design of human performance systems. *Journal of Organizational Behavior Management, 9,* 125–129. https://doi.org/10.1300/J075v09n01_09

McGee, H. M., & Crowley-Koch, B. J. (2021). Performance assessment of organizations. *Journal of Organizational Behavior Management, 41*(3), 255–285. https://doi. org/10.1080/01608061.2021.1909687

Parmenter, D. (2015). *Key performance indicators: Developing, implementing, and using winning KPIs* (3rd ed.). John Wiley & Sons.

Silbaugh, B. C., & El Fattal, R. (2022). Exploring quality in the applied behavior analysis service delivery industry. *Behavior Analysis in Practice, 15*, 571–590. https://doi. org/10.1007/s40617-021-00627-y

Silbaugh, B. C. (2023). Discussion and conceptual analysis of four group contingencies for behavioral process improvement in an ABA service delivery quality framework. *Behavior Analysis in Practice, 16*, 421–436. https://doi.org/10.1007/ s40617-022-00750-4

Skinner, B. F. (1974). *About behaviorism.* Random House, Inc.

5 Benefits of Quality Control

Imagine that you are a BCBA supervising the autism care team for a 5-year-old-boy with autism and your team provides those services in-home. We will call the patient Craig. Craig receives 35 hours per week of ABA therapy and two RBTs provide his direct treatment. It's Monday morning and you have a supervision session scheduled for 8:30 am. On your way to the patient's home, you get a call from the scheduler that the RBT got a flat tire and they are working on finding a sub. Ten minutes pass and you are halfway to the patient's home. You receive a call from the scheduler and its good news—the other RBT on the case is available to sub and they will arrive approximately at the same time you do.

Finally, you arrive at Craig's home and the sub beat you there and has already started session. You haven't been out to see Craig for a week and you are eager to see how a few of the new behavioral interventions are going. But when you walk into Craig's home, his dad pulls you aside to discuss a new behavioral concern. Craig has been voiding all over the house! Ten minutes pass, you thank dad for letting you know of the issue and explain that you will circle back to the issue at your next parent support session.

Okay, finally you make your way upstairs to Craig's room where the session is under way. But the moment you enter the room, greet the RBT, and open your laptop, you receive a Google Chat message from the clinical director announcing its Jasmine's birthday! Woo hoo! Okay, that's great, but you are trying to focus on your session!

As you log into the online data collection system you check in with the RBT. She shares that she worked with a client yesterday who "went into crisis" and the RBT shows you the scratches and bite marks on her arm. You sympathize with her, but you also REALLY need to see her run the session so you can start observing how things are going. So, you ask her to please proceed and to run the new intraverbal target you introduced last week. Unfortunately, she did not realize that the target was created in the baseline section of Craig's program and has not implemented it yet. Ugh! No data? A week went by and it just feels like a waste. Time flies by and it's time to give Craig

DOI: 10.4324/9781003475095-5

a 15-minute break, and your chance to see the intraverbal target implemented by your RBT and assess procedural fidelity, is gone.

Highly Practical and Efficient

This hypothetical but very realistic scenario represents how incredibly difficult case supervision of ABA autism service programs can be. In the midst of all this chaos, distractions, and competing contingencies, how in the world is a BCBA supervisor supposed to write, oversee, monitor, and systematically adjust behavioral interventions in the evidence-based practice of ABA, and assess procedural fidelity and interobserver agreement? Studies show that researchers can assess interobserver agreement and procedural fidelity, so why can't practitioners?

In universities around the world where ABA research is conducted, researchers have the luxury of assessing procedural fidelity and interobserver agreement from video recordings of sessions, between sessions, in the comfort of their distraction-free labs or home offices. For example, if the researcher is conducting an ABA research study in a participant's home, they can visit the participant, run 5–10 five-minute sessions of a single behavioral intervention, video record those sessions, return to the lab, write a highly detailed procedural fidelity assessment checklist, slowly and gradually watch and re-watch the videos, and collect trial-by-trial data on the research assistant's implementation of the behavioral intervention, one intervention component (e.g., SD, prompt, reinforcement contingency, reinforcer duration, magnitude of reinforcement) at a time. This approach to assessing procedural fidelity with any kind of regularity in clinical practice is absolutely impossible because of all of the BCBA's competing contingencies in the context where interventions occur, and because the BCBA often has dozens of behavioral interventions programmed and being run by RBTs.

The approach described in the current model is highly practical and efficient because it requires no video recording, no individualized data sheets, and can be completed within ten minutes for any skill acquisition target anywhere, any time. And documentation is straightforward and simple. Even in the chaos of sessions like Craig's, the clinical BCBA can squeeze in a ten-minute quality control cycle. I know because I have done it, time and time again!

Improves Target Data Quality

The BCBA supervisors rely, among other things, on graphed behavior data to make clinical decisions for their clients. Decisions based on graphed data are only as good as the data! Variability in graphed behavioral data could represent changes in patient behavior, data collection errors or drift, or drift in the accurate implementation of behavioral interventions. Bad clinical decisions can lead to the implementation of ineffective behavioral interventions, or worse, interventions that worsen behavior! Clients have a right to effective behavioral treatment (Van Houten et al., 1988). That's why it is essential that BCBA supervisors conduct quality control cycles on behavioral interventions routinely.

Quality control cycles improve target data quality through procedural fidelity assessment, interobserver agreement assessment, and problem solving to resolve discrepancies between implementation and the quality plan. Consistent implementation of quality control cycles over time should correspond with improvements in the quality of graphed behavioral data and as a result improve the BCBA's ability to make data-based decisions that enhance treatment effectiveness. For example, as the BCBA supervisor systematically manipulates independent variables across phases and conditions, they should begin to see reductions in variability about the data paths, increasing trends in the desired direction of behavior change, and fewer trials needed to meet mastery criteria.

Reduces Risk of False Positive Target Mastery

All too commonly I have come across ABA autism service organizations that employ BCBA supervisors who are rushed, pressured, and cajoled to introduce large numbers of behavior-change programs for individual patients (e.g., 30–40 skill acquisition and behavior-reduction targets for one client, all at once). Pressuring BCBA supervisors in this way can result in total neglect of procedural fidelity and interobserver agreement. This pressure can spread downstream to the RBT, such as in the form of excessive and inappropriate expectations for daily trial counts per target. If you introduce 30–40 targets at once, and pressure your RBT to run 20 trials per target per day, please stop. If your clinical director or manager is pressuring you to put that kind of pressure on your RBT, please stop. Not only does this highly inappropriate clinical practice ignore the fact that there is only so much reinforcement to spread across a day for discrete trial training and natural environment teaching and therefore occasions higher rates of challenging patient behavior, but it also creates the conditions in which BCBA-RBT dyads toss their skeptic hats in the trash and assume every so-called mastered target is really mastered.

Quality control cycles solve this problem. Use the model in this book to conduct quality control cycles and do not master out a target until your team demonstrates high procedural fidelity and high interobserver agreement. Put another way, you can use quality control over BIQ to minimize and prevent false positive target mastery.

Facilitates Collaboration Between BCBA and RBT

Many RBTs have told me time and time again that they have experienced BCBA supervisors who stop by the session, greet them, spend the bulk of their time with their face buried in their laptop, then tell them that they're doing great and promptly leave without providing training, authentic support, or constructive feedback. I have also heard from many RBTs, stories of clinical BCBA supervisors who show up to session, bark out commands and expect compliance from the RBT without question, and refuse to answer the RBT's questions or skirt around their questions. But RBTs need and want support, training, coaching, advising, mentorship, other forms of professional development, and collaboration.

A major benefit of routinely conducting quality control cycles is collaboration between the BCBA and RBT. At the end of each quality control cycle when the data are discussed, the BCBA and RBT problem solve together and talk about the components of the behavioral intervention that were implemented correctly, those that were not, and opportunities to clarify the protocol or other adjustments they can make in the environment to improve the intervention's implementation, which may also include simplifying the intervention. This conversation is a great opportunity for BCBAs to hear what the RBT has to say, to learn from their observations and experience, and to design behavioral interventions that are not only effective for the patient but acceptable and feasible for the RBT.

Reduces RBT Burnout

It is difficult to provide high-quality services when employees burn out, and leave. Burnout can be defined as, "a syndrome of emotional exhaustion, depersonalization, and reduced personal accomplishment that can occur among individuals who work with people in some capacity" (Maslach et al., 1996, p. 4). In ABA service delivery, emotional exhaustion, depersonalization, and feeling a lack of personal accomplishment may lead to ethics code violations, high turnover (e.g., Kazemi et al., 2015), and low life and work satisfaction (Kranak, 2022).

Plantiveau et al. (2018) suggest that burnout results from chronic exposure to stress on-the-job and that burnout in the industry may pose a significant public health problem. In their recent study, 183 behavior analytic professionals (i.e., RBT®, BCaBA®, BCBA®, BCBA-D®, and students) completed a survey on demographics, job satisfaction, and burnout using the Maslach burnout inventory. Only 52% of respondents reported being satisfied with their work conditions. Roughly a fourth of respondents scored within the high emotional exhaustion range, roughly a third scored high on depersonalization, and 50% scored high on lack of accomplishment. The researchers note that their data contrast with prior studies of RBT®s and burnout; however, it is important to note those studies were published between 2009 and 2014 and therefore may be unrepresentative of the current industry.

In a survey study by Slowiak and DeLongchamp (2022), 826 ABA practitioners who responded to recruitment messages via professional organizations,

Listservs, and social media pages; answered questions on topics including self-care strategies, work engagement, and burnout (i.e., using the 16-item Oldenburg Burnout Inventory). Similar to the findings of Plantiveau et al., moderate-to-high levels of burnout were reported by 72% of respondents. Burnout of BCBAs and RBTs is likely a pervasive problem that may have been magnified by the COVID-19 pandemic (e.g., Jimenez-Gomez et al., 2021).

Some studies suggest perceived supervisor support is negatively associated with burnout. In one study, perceived supervisor support was associated with lower burnout in behavior technicians who worked in ABA schools in Ireland (Gibson et al., 2009), and in another study a similar finding was found in behavior technicians who provided in-home services in the United States (Hurt et al., 2013). In a report to the Florida Developmental Disabilities Council, Gravina and colleagues (2023) described a qualitative study they conducted with focus groups of 14 RBTs and 24 BCBAs to better understand how current working conditions, challenges faced in clinical practice, and available training, are related to the behavior-therapist shortage in Florida. In both groups, a common theme that emerged was a perceived adverse impact of supervision support or quality on RBT burnout, especially in service of individuals who engaged in challenging behavior and/or adults.

Many of the variables that research suggests are predictive of burnout and turnover, such as satisfactory training, supervision, and pay (Kazemi et al., 2015); opportunities for advancement and praise for good work (Kazemi et al., 2015); and reinforcement for engaging in self-care and health-promoting activities (e.g., Slowiak & DeLongchamp, 2022); can be engineered into ABA service delivery processing systems when managers for quality have the right tools (e.g., Luke et al., 2024), resources, and support from leadership.

My personal experience using the current model to control BIQ is that it probably reduces RBT burnout by providing what a sample of RBT survey respondents in Florida asked for more of in the workplace (Gravina et al., 2023): increased frequency and quality of supportive and constructive feedback on performance, clearer expectations (i.e., implement the protocol and collect data as written), improved communication and rapport, increased consistency of supervision practices, being more present during observations, and opportunities to provide supervisors with feedback. Studies are needed to evaluate the relationship between quality control over BIQ and burnout, to empirically determine whether implementation of higher quality BIQ reduces self-reported stress on-the-job, intentions to quit, and scores on assessments of burnout; and increased self-reported work satisfaction.

Chapter Summary

Clinical BCBA supervisors face many challenges and competing contingencies during supervision sessions, all of which can serve as barriers to controlling BIQ. The current model of quality control over BIQ can help BCBAs overcome those barriers and offers numerous benefits. The BCBAs can complete a single quality control cycle in under ten minutes for any skill acquisition protocol anywhere, anytime. Accordingly, the current model is both highly practical and efficient. The model reduces variability in graphs of behavior data by eliminating variability associated with implementation of the independent variable and data collection accuracy. By reducing those sources of variability, the current model reduces the risk of false positive mastery of acquisition targets. Feedback and problem solving between successive cycles improves collaboration between the BCBA and RBT. Lastly, the current model may reduce RBT burnout and thus turnover by increasing the frequency quality of supportive and constructive feedback on performance, clearer expectations for the RBT, improved communication, more consistent supervision practices, a more engaged presence during observations, and opportunities to give supervisors constructive feedback that results in the clarification or revision of behavioral intervention protocols.

References

Gibson, J. A., Grey, I. M., & Hastings, R. P. (2009). Supervisor support as a predictor of burnout and therapeutic self-efficacy in therapists working in ABA schools. *Journal of Autism Developmental Disorders, 39*(7), 1024–1030. https://doi.org/10.1007/s10803-009-0709-4

Gravina, N., Leon, Y., Peters, K., Bacotti, J., McGarry, K., & Nastasi, J. (2023). *Understanding the behavior therapist shortage in Florida.* Florida Developmental Disabilities Council, Inc. https://fddc.org/wp-content/uploads/2023/10/Addressing-the-Behavior-Therapist-Shortage-Final-Report.pdf

Hurt, A. A., Grist, C. L., Malesky, L. A., & McCord, D. M. (2013). Personality traits associated with occupational 'burnout' in ABA therapists. *Journal of Applied Research in Intellectual Disabilities, 26*, 299–308. https://doi.org/10.1111/jar.12043

Jimenez-Gomez, C., Sawhney, G., & Albert, K. M. (2021). Impact of COVID-19 on the applied behavior analysis workforce: Comparison across remote and nonremote workers. *Behavior Analysis in Practice, 14*, 873–882. https://doi.org/10.1007/s40617-021-00625-0

Kazemi, E., Shapiro, M., & Kavner, A. (2015). Predictors of intention to turnover in behavior technicians working with individuals with autism spectrum disorder. *Research in Autism Spectrum Disorders, 17*, 106–115. https://doi.org/10.1016/j.rasd.2015.06.012

Kranak, M. P. (2022). Put out the fire before it spreads: On equipping behavior analysts with strategies to mitigate burnout. *Behavior Analysis: Research and Practice, 22*(4), 404–406. https://doi.org/10.1037/bar0000255

Luke, M. M., Dams, P., & Lichtenberger, S. N. (2024). Improving human-service organizations through process mapping: A tutorial for practitioners. *Behavior Analysis in Practice.* https://doi.org/10.1007/s40617-024-00906-4

Maslach, C., Jackson, S. E., & Leiter, M. P. (1996). *Maslach burnout inventory manual.* Consulting Psychologists Press.

Plantiveau, C., Dounavi, K., & Virues-Ortega, J. (2018). High levels of burnout among early-career board-certified behavior analysts with low collegial support in the work environment. *European Journal of Behavior Analysis, 19*(2), 195–207. https://doi.org/10.1080/15021149.2018.1438339

Slowiak, J. M., & DeLongchamp, A. C. (2022). Self-care strategies and job-crafting practices among behavior analysts: Do they predict perceptions of work-life balance, work engagement, and burnout? *Behavior Analysis in Practice, 15*(2), 414–432. https://doi.org/10.1007/s40617-021-00570-y

Van Houten, R., Axelrod, S., Bailey, J. S., Favell, J. E., Foxx, R. M., Iwata, B. A., & Lovaas, O. I. (1988). The right to effective behavioral treatment. *Journal of Applied Behavior Analysis, 21*(4), 381–384. https://doi.org/10.1901/jaba.1988.21-381

6 Troubleshooting and Reducing Barriers

Establishing a routine process for controlling BIQ is a major accomplishment in any ABA autism service organization. But it will not always be easy. While integrating this new cultural practice into your current clinical practice as a BCBA, your BCBAs' clinical practices as a quality manager or clinical director, or throughout your organizations at scale as a leader in a position of power, there will be barriers to overcome. You will encounter tough problems along the way, but the troubleshooting steps and tips in this chapter can help you overcome them, one at a time. Make sure to celebrate every single barrier overcome and problem solved!

As BCBA-RBT dyads repeatedly engage in quality control, the incidence of quality control cycles will vary, as will the outcomes of quality control cycles. What if variability in quality control practices increase or becomes unstable over time? What if variability in quality control cycle outcomes vary widely or become unstable over time? What if BCBA-RBT dyads are hesitant to engage in this practice routinely under your management?

Quality control over BIQ is a cultural practice. Cultural practice variability is under antecedent and consequent stimulus control. Reducing variability in any cultural practice requires attention paid to the environment where it occurs and modifying antecedents and consequences until you obtain the desired result. This chapter offers some suggestions for troubleshooting barriers to conducting quality control cycles and controlling variability in quality control cycle outcomes though modifications of antecedents and consequences targeting specific BCBA and RBT repertoires at each step of a quality control cycle. It will be particularly helpful to BCBA supervisors and quality managers to revisit this chapter periodically for the first year or so that they apply the current model to control BIQ.

Step 1. Initiate a Quality Control Cycle

The first step of engaging in a quality control cycle is the BCBA or RBT asks their colleague to conduct one. For new BCBA-RBT dyads, the BCBA trains

DOI: 10.4324/9781003475095-6

the RBT how to conduct quality control cycles, so BCBA initiations of quality control cycles exert stronger antecedent stimulus control over RBT participation than other stimuli in the clinical context. Quality control outcomes are influenced by the frequency that quality control cycles occur. The BIQ can be expected to increase with increases in the incidence of quality control cycles. The quality of a client's behavioral interventions should be sampled and controlled frequently enough to ensure that the BCBA-RBT dyad can consistently control the quality of their behavioral interventions. You often cannot sample the quality of all targets every session, so BIQ should be sampled frequently enough to obtain data that are representative of the quality of a client's behavioral interventions overall.

Engaging in quality control over BIQ is only one of the BCBA's many responsibilities in a supervision or protocol modification session. Entering a supervision session for a BCBA is like arriving at a buffet. Concurrently arranged reinforcement is everywhere. Buffets have numerous dishes to choose from, and you might want to try everything, but you can only put so much food on your plate at once. As someone famous (I forgot whom) once said, you can have it all, but you can't have it all at the same time. Something has to give. When a BCBA walks into a supervision session, they may want to tackle all of their responsibilities. And they often can. But not all at the same time. To conduct a quality control cycle, the BCBA has to put everything else aside for roughly ten minutes. Multi-tasking will not cut it! Here are seven tips for increasing the initiation of quality control cycles.

Tip 1: Cycle Starter Phrases

For some new BCBA-RBT dyads, it will feel very natural for the BCBA to walk into a supervision session and ask their RBT to conduct a quality control cycle. For other dyads, it might feel uncomfortable. When it is uncomfortable, it might be hard to find the words to say to initiate the cycle.

When the BCBA and RBT are piloting the process for the first time it is probably helpful if the BCBA first provides a rationale for conducting a quality control cycle and then explains the difference between independent-variable and dependent-variable integrity. After the explanation, the BCBA can say something like, "Would you like to start with the IV or the DV?".

After the BCBA-RBT dyad has some experience conducting quality control cycles together, the BCBA may encounter wide variability in how quickly RBTs become fluent in the language of quality control cycles as described in this book. For example, some RBTs will quickly acquire intraverbal responses "IV" "DV" in response to questions about which kind of quality control cycle they want to initiate, while others will take longer to learn to discriminate between IV and DV quality control cycles. Here are some suggestions for phrasing that BCBAs can use over time to initiate cycles and account for that learning curve. The BCBAs can keep a quality control cheat sheet on their laptop computer and access the cheat sheet as a job aide with the following quality cycle starters:

- "Let's take a look at how you are teaching this. We call that IV integrity or procedural fidelity."
- "We can check how you are teaching this target, or we can check data collection. Which do you prefer?"
- "We can check how you are teaching it to make sure I wrote the protocol clearly. Or we can see if we collect the same data. Which should we try first?"
- "The IV is about how accurate you are teaching the target, and the DV is your client's response. Which do you want to check first?"
- "The IV is the intervention protocol and the DV is the learner's response. Which do you want to look at first?"
- "The target instructions are the independent variable or intervention. When you collect data on your client's responses, you are measuring the DV or dependent variable. Perhaps we start with the independent variable?"
- "Your client's responses are the dependent variable. Their responses depend on the extent to which you implement the intervention as it is written here (pointing to the target on a tablet). Would you like me to assess the accuracy of your implementation, or the accuracy of your data collection?"

When the BCBA-RBT dyad have completed roughly 20–30 quality control cycles, a job aide for cycle starter phrasing should no longer be needed by the BCBA to easily and quickly initiate quality control cycles, and they should move to more direct, clear, and efficient language such as,

- "Shall we do a QC check on the IV, DV, or both?"
  or
- "Would you like to do a QC on the IV or the DV?".

Tip 2: BCBA Checklist

Checklists may be helpful to increase BCBA-initiated quality control cycles. To ensure they initiate at least one quality control cycle, it may be helpful for the BCBA to prepare a checklist before their supervision session. For in-home service providers, the BCBA may arrive early at their session, hang out in their car, and write down a checklist of five things that they are going to accomplish in the session. For example, the BCBA might write down that they are going to (1) make a list of materials and supplies that the RBT is in need of, (2) collect current data on toileting from the caregiver, (3) write a behavior reduction target in the data collection system for hand mouthing, (4) conduct a quality control cycle on the new play skills target, and (5) complete an assessment for the client's pending reauthorization due in two weeks.

When the BCBA enters the home, they should have the checklist out so it can serve as an antecedent stimulus (i.e., a temporary job aide in this case) that increases the likelihood that they will complete not only the quality control cycle but also their other tasks. In the event that they encounter potential distractions, they may be more prepared to dodge, duck, dive, and dip their way around those distractions like a game a dodgeball and get the job done.

Tip 3: Alarms

Alarms represent another option. These are helpful for RBTs to initiate more quality control cycles. RBTs can use company-issued tablets to access their clients' programs and collect behavior data. Tablets have alarm applications that can be set up to prompt RBTs to complete certain tasks, including quality control cycles.

Tip 4: Session Checklist

Another common practice is for ABA sessions to be structured with a session checklist. A session checklist is a list of structural elements of the session or tasks that the RBT is expected to complete before the session ends. For example, tasks may include giving the client a break every 2 hours, inviting a caregiver to participate in session, organizing the toy bin, and sanitizing the toys and instructional materials. Session checklists may increase the likelihood that RBTs initiate quality control cycles during supervision sessions. To increase the likelihood the RBT will initiate a quality control cycle, it may be helpful to add "initiate quality control cycle" to the session checklist. However, note that it is important that contingencies are arranged to ensure that the RBTs complete their session checklist. It is often not enough to simply have the checklist accessible. Direct treatment sessions too are like buffets for RBTs. Only so much can fit on their plate at once.

Tip 5: Internal Chat Prompts

Another option to use is text-based prompting via internal group chat applications such as Google Chat®. This approach can help RBTs and BCBAs conduct more quality control cycles. For example, an organization can use Google Chat® "space" and "chat" options for communicating within and across departments throughout the workday. Everyone in the company, including RBTs, can be logged into the chat app and can receive and send messages throughout the day. Each client can have a "space" with their autism care team members associated with the space. If an RBT has a question, they can post it on their client's space to the rest of the autism care team, or they can directly message a colleague or supervisor. The director of clinical quality, a clinical director, a manager for quality, or someone with similar responsibilities but a different title, should be a member of all clients' spaces too. They can use the app to prompt autism care teams to conduct quality control cycles either individually, by group, or department-wide. This approach may be especially helpful for a given autism-care team when one specific team member (i.e., a particular RBT or BCBA) initiates too few quality control cycles.

Tip 6: BCBA Delays to Feedback

This technique can be used to increase initiations of quality control cycles by RBTs by loosening antecedent stimulus control over quality control cycle initiations by the BCBA. The RBTs expect BCBAs to initiate conversation, make observations, and give feedback on RBT performance. If BCBA feedback on RBT performance is reinforcing, the passage of time without feedback from the BCBA within session may function as an establishing operation for mands from the RBT to engage in practices, such as quality control cycles, that produce BCBA feedback. To use this technique, the BCBA merely sits back, observes the RBT, and waits until the RBT mands for a quality control cycle. Contingent on the mand the BCBA can agree to complete the quality control cycle, engage in the practice, and provide positive reinforcement to the RBT in the form of (a) descriptive praise for the components of the behavioral intervention they implemented correctly and (b) corrective feedback that helps the RBT implement the intervention with higher BIQ in the next cycle.

Tip 7. Remote Micro-Supervision Sessions

A major barrier to conducting quality control cycles for all BCBAs is the availability of time to spend with their RBTs and clients. For example, often the time a BCBA can spend in supervision sessions for a given client per week is often limited to the quantity of supervision hours authorized by an insurance company for the service period. If services are provided in-home or in the community (as opposed to center-based service delivery), BCBAs have to work extra hard to minimize their drive time between the office, their home, clients' homes, and community settings where services are delivered. Fortunately, since the COVID-19 pandemic, remote supervision via videoconference applications has become a more accessible option for BCBAs. Practice parameters for delivering ABA services via telehealth are available from CASP online (CASP, n.d.). When payors do not prohibit this modality of supervision, BCBAs can use it to reduce or eliminate commute time and maximize their time spent with RBTs and clients. Remote supervision as a modality of service delivery provides the BCBA with the ability to use brief, targeted, remote micro-supervision sessions to conduct quality control cycles.

A remote micro-supervision session is loosely defined here as a relatively brief impromptu supervision session initiated by a BCBA or an RBT in which only one supervisory task is performed, such as quality control over BIQ, for a duration of less than 30 minutes. Applications like Google Chat® and Google Space® have a feature that enables any employee in the chat or space to initiate a remote supervision session via the videoconference application Google Meet®. My preference is to conduct as much supervision in-person as possible. However, when an organization hires new staff or onboards new clients, it can place a strain on supervision for BCBAs involved in those processes. The strain can be alleviated by shifting more supervision time from in-person to remote. Under those conditions, the BCBA can maintain quality control over BIQ by spontaneously initiating brief remote supervision sessions via Google Meet® to conduct one or more quality control cycles.

A simple hypothetical scenario will illustrate. Mira is an RBT who provides ABA therapy to Ben, a 5-year-old boy with autism, in his home, for ten hours per week, two hours per day. Her BCBA clinical supervisor is named Krista. This morning, Krista was scheduled to conduct an assessment for a new client, which placed a strain on her ability to commute to Ben's home for Mira's supervision today. To compensate, Krista messages Mira in the chat, "Good morning Mira! I hoped to stop by for supervision this morning but I'm also scheduled for a new client assessment this afternoon. Preparing for the assessment will take longer than expected, so I won't make it out to Ben's home. Could I drop in via Google Meet for 20 minutes to check in on a few things and conduct a QC? Any target of your choice!". A few minutes later Mira responds in the chat, "I totally understand. Yes, that would be great. I want to do a QC on the handwashing target because I'm not sure if I'm prompt fading correctly. I'll send you the Google Meet link. What time?". Krista immediately responds, "8:30am. Thanks Mira!". At 8:30am, Krista and Mira jump into the Google Meet room, touch base on a few things to support Mira for the day, and conduct two quality control cycles, all within a 20-minute remote supervision session. The outcome of the first quality control cycle completed for procedural fidelity was 85%, and the outcome improved with the second cycle at 100%. Krista completes her clinical documentation after the supervision session and begins to prepare for her assessment. Quality control practices were maintained, Krista feels accomplished, and Mira feels supported and empowered to run her session without additional supervision that day. And not a moment was spent on BCBA or RBT practices that do not benefit the client.

Step 2. Select a Target

Targets are generally introduced either remotely (i.e., outside of direct treatment sessions) or during supervision of a direct treatment session. BCBAs are probably more likely to introduce a completely new skill acquisition target without the RBT's knowledge when they program it remotely. When quality control cycles are new to BCBA-RBT dyads, generally the quality plan is not met for a new skill acquisition target and the RBT requires training to establish discriminative stimulus control over their intervention practices by the target protocol.

If a skill acquisition target was introduced remotely, the RBT may have had a chance to practice it before the BCBA arrives for supervision to conduct the first quality control cycle on that target. In that circumstance, the BCBA should initiate and conduct a quality control cycle on that target in the next supervision session. Alternatively, if the RBT did not have a chance to practice before the BCBA arrives, it is recommended that rather than conduct a quality control cycle, the dyad discuss the target, role-play or give the RBT the benefit of observing the BCBA model the behavioral intervention, and then conduct a quality control cycle later in that session or in the next supervision session. The advantage of this approach is that the BCBA-RBT dyad can avoid that sudden unpleasant feeling that the quality control cycle is pointless within one or two trials into the cycle because the RBT is implementing most steps incorrectly or has lots of questions. This approach also helps ensure the BCBA provides the necessary training to their RBTs before asking them to implement an intervention during a quality control cycle they simply are not ready for.

Skill acquisition targets introduced or programmed during a supervision session can be completed solely by the BCBA, or through collaboration between the BCBA and the RBT. When a new target is introduced solely by the BCBA, take the same approach described earlier for targets introduced remotely. However, for skill acquisition targets programmed collaboratively, BCBA-RBT dyads may be comfortable jumping right into a quality control cycle.

Step 3. Protocol Review

Protocol review sometimes results in the BCBA-RBT dyad catching errors in the behavioral intervention protocol such as typos, missing information, or excess information that distract from or function as barriers to the RBT's implementation coming under strong discriminative stimulus control by the intervention protocol. For example, perhaps the schedule of reinforcement was written incorrectly, the BCBA used an unfamiliar acronym, or major intervention protocol components are missing (e.g., the prompt fading procedure and discriminative stimuli are unspecified). If the dyad discovers these issues during protocol review, I recommend the BCBA and RBT stop the cycle, and instead collaborate to revise and improve the protocol instructions.

Once errors in a behavioral intervention protocol have been corrected, the BCBA-RBT dyad should conduct quality control over that behavioral intervention in a subsequent session to ensure that the RBT's implementation of the intervention during the quality control cycle on that target reflects discriminative stimulus control over their performance by the protocol instructions, not by the BCBA's verbal behavior emitted during collaboration. Simply said, to make sure what you are seeing during the observation portion of the cycle is a result of the protocol the RBT read, not something you said; thereby enabling the RBT to implement the protocol with high procedural fidelity and collect accurate data consistently, in your absence.

Similarly, for BCBAs early into the process of conducting quality control, some RBTs will show a tendency to ask for clarification or additional information at the review stage. Answering the RBT's questions at the review stage puts them at a disadvantage. It poses a risk to the internal validity of the quality control cycle if the RBT's performance becomes dually influenced by the BCBA's answers to the RBT's questions and the protocol. Discussion of the intervention protocol details between the BCBA and RBT can also really drag out the process and adversely impact efficiency. High-performing BCBA-RBT dyads do not discuss the protocol during this stage. If the BCBA is strict and consistent about this particular practice, most RBTs will learn to solicit feedback in the analysis step of the cycle instead of the problematic practice of asking for information at the start of the cycle and preventing the BCBA from discovering performance errors and faulty stimulus control over implementation by the written protocol. For RBTs to consistently implement high-quality behavioral interventions as a result of engaging in quality control cycles, feedback identifying inevitable errors in implementation needs to become conditioned positive reinforcement for their participation—and feedback as differential reinforcement contingent on implementing quality control cycles solely in response to the intervention protocol, is how you do it!

When I first started to conduct quality control cycles, I noted more variability in BIQ across cycles than expected. To troubleshoot, I started to more closely examine how I wrote my targets. This process brought to my attention that there was perhaps too much variability in how I wrote my targets. For example, for some RBTs but not others, I wrote out specific instructions for how to collect data on certain targets. Or for some targets but not others, I explicitly stated the prompt fading strategy. And for some targets, I specified the SD in the protocol before I specified the schedule of reinforcement or data-collection procedures, but for other targets I specified the schedule of reinforcement before specifying the SD. Sometimes, I used acronyms in my protocols that my RBTs were unfamiliar with (and of course they did not tell me—they just guessed at the acronym and ran the target!). All that is to say that my protocol writing was inconsistent, and I used terminology or acronyms with weak discriminative stimulus control over RBTs' quality-plan implementation.

To reduce variability in BIQ due to variability in how protocols are written, I highly recommend adopting a standard protocol writing format that includes specific intervention components that are always specified (e.g., discriminative stimulus, target response, intertrial interval, reinforcer parameters, reinforcer schedule, prompt fading strategy, setting or context) for all targets, and the use of a standard set of ABA terms (i.e., jargon). As BCBA-RBT dyads complete repeated quality control cycles across multiple exemplars of standardized protocol templates, I believe RBTs acquire what I consider the holy grail of RBT protocol implementation repertoires: a generalized behavioral intervention protocol implementation repertoire characterized by implementing any new behavioral intervention protocol without additional training, at 80% or higher procedural fidelity.

Step 4. Select Procedural Fidelity, Interobserver Agreement, or Both

In my experience, high interobserver agreement is easier to attain than high procedural fidelity, and therefore requires lower rates of quality control cycles to maintain. However, if obtaining good outcomes (i.e., 90% interobserver agreement) from quality control cycles is reinforcing, then temporarily shifting to a higher ratio of interobserver agreement (i.e., dependent variable integrity) to procedural fidelity (i.e., independent variable integrity) quality control cycles (e.g., three interobserver agreement to every one procedural fidelity) may accelerate the incidence of quality control over BIQ. In the same way that you might intersperse maintenance or easy tasks with skill acquisition or harder tasks, or build momentum with a high-probability instructional sequence (Mace et al., 1988) to increase the rate of responding for clients; interspersal of interobserver agreement cycles with procedural fidelity cycles, or building momentum with multiple interobserver agreement cycles before each procedural fidelity cycle, may increase the rate of quality control cycles and improve outcomes. However, be careful to strike a balance that avoids neglecting procedural fidelity. Do not attempt to assess interobserver agreement and procedural fidelity concurrently in a quality control cycle until your dyad is fluent in the process.

Step 5. Define the Observation Period

At this step, the BCBA and RBT decide how many trials to run, or how long the observation period will be. The more trials you run and the longer you observe the RBT implement the behavioral intervention, the more time it takes to conduct a quality control cycle and the less likely you are to fit it into the session on a given day. During supervision sessions in which there are fewer competing contingencies, consider getting a more representative sample of the quality of behavioral intervention implementation by running 10 or more trials per cycle, or running cycles for five or more minutes. During supervision sessions in which you are crunched for time, consider running five trials per cycle or observing for two-minute observation periods.

Step 6. RBT Initiates Implementation

It is not productive for RBTs to initiate quality control cycles at motivationally suboptimal times for their clients. RBTs who effectively implement skill acquisition targets learn to identify the presence and absence of establishing operations (e.g., Michael, 2004) for positive reinforcement needed to teach skills (e.g., intraverbals and play skills) before they teach them. For example, for early learners (e.g., children aged 2 to 5 years) I have always taught my RBTs to wait for the client to reach, look toward, follow, or otherwise observably initiate towards the RBT before teaching a target because the initiation is an observable indicator of an establishing operation for positive reinforcement (I learned that practice early in my career from Coyne & Associates in southern California back in 2008). Today practitioners might call that initiation a form of "assent" (e.g., Linnehan et al., 2023). Often establishing operations for negative reinforcement can be manipulated instantly for their behavior-altering effects and the RBT can immediately implement the behavioral intervention, such as functional communication training for escape maintained challenging behavior (Carr & Durand, 1985) or non-removal of the spoon to treat food refusal in pediatric feeding disorders (e.g., Silbaugh et al., 2018). However, for some clients, the RBT may need to follow their lead for a few minutes, or longer, to capture an establishing operation for positive reinforcement. If the RBT feels rushed, the intervention will feel forced, and their performance is likely to differ from how they perform with the client under less time-pressured conditions. The learner is also likely to respond to intervention differently than they otherwise would if the RBT properly captured their motivation first. Thus, at this step of the quality control cycle, it is helpful for the BCBA to relieve pressure on the RBT to perform by encouraging them to take their time to follow the client's lead and establish motivation before starting to teach. Sometimes, the way I do this is to tell the RBT, "No rush. Find your groove first, and when he is motivated, that's the best time to start".

Step 7. Implementation and Observation Period

Are you hesitant to give feedback in-the-moment? Or are you more inclined to correct your RBTs' performance when you see it and shower your RBTs with praise for desired performance throughout the session? If you are the latter, like me, this next suggestion is especially important. The implementation and observation period is your only opportunity in the cycle to see how the RBT implements the intervention in response to the protocol you have written. The more trials the RBT conducts, or the longer you observe, the more likely you are to get a representative sample of their performance. If you notice early into the observation period that procedural fidelity is low, you may feel the need to correct their performance immediately. If you notice instead that their implementation of the intervention is perfect and the learner is happy and responding well to treatment, you may feel the urge to join your RBT in praising the learner, or praise the RBT for their outstanding performance. Either way, you would be interfering with the process and diminishing the internal validity of the quality control process by introducing extraneous variables (e.g., BCBA stimulus control) which could introduce variability into the quality control outcome. Don't do it. Your RBT and the client are doing a dance.

The learner initiates to the RBT, the RBT delivers an SD, and the learner responds. The RBT delivers feedback. Stimuli are re-arranged. The learner initiates to the RBT, the RBT delivers an SD, and the learner responds. The RBT delivers feedback, and functionally interdependent interactions between the RBT and the learner continue until the end of the observation period. Douglas Greer calls this interlocking interaction between teacher and learner, a "learn unit", and the learn unit a fundamental of pedagogy (Greer & McDonough, 1999). In a learn unit, the RBT and client engage in behaviors that serve as controlling antecedents and consequences for each other's behavior. In other words, their behaviors are interlocked by contingencies of reinforcement. In the current model of quality control over behavioral interventions it is assumed that BCBA and RBT interactions occurring during the observation period disrupt the interlocks that constitute learn units and as a result disrupts the discriminative stimulus control over the RBT's involvement in the interlock by the intervention protocol. Observe for the full duration of the observation period or the total number of trials agreed upon in advance, and only then give them feedback. Let them dance.

Step 8. Analysis

In this step, the BCBA-RBT dyad discuss the outcome of the quality control cycle and engage in collaborative problem solving to increase procedural fidelity or interobserver agreement. Variability in quality control attributable to this step of the process can come from multiple sources, including but not limited to how the BCBA delivers feedback and how the RBT responds to feedback.

BCBA Feedback Delivery

At the start of the discussion, the BCBA estimates procedural fidelity or calculates interobserver agreement, and gives the RBT feedback on their performance. As Ehrlich et al. (2020) noted, feedback has been broadly defined in our field as, "information about a performance that allows the individual to change his or her behavior" (Daniels & Daniels, 2006, p. 171). Feedback is the verbal behavior of one person with the potential to exert influence on another person's behavior through antecedent or consequent stimulus control.

Based on that idea, Erlich et al. (2020) suggest that "feedback might function as a motivating operation and establish instructional rules about discriminated-operant performance or alter the effects of certain environmental variables" (p. 20) on the receiving employee's behavior. Thus, how the BCBA delivers feedback in the analysis step of a quality control cycle may contribute to variability in the RBT's implementation of the quality plan. The purpose of the feedback is to maintain the RBT's high-quality implementation of the behavioral intervention (i.e., the quality plan) or to improve implementation in the future.

There are different types of feedback used in the workplace. In my opinion, the most effective and acceptable feedback a BCBA can give an RBT in a quality control cycle is corrective or affirming, positive, and optimistic. Erlich et al. (2023) defined corrective feedback as, "the delivery of information to an individual in a manner that changes or reduces a specific response or response class" (p. 19). Reid and colleagues (2012) defined positive or supportive feedback as, "information about the quality of work that includes approval or praise" (p. 114). Here optimistic feedback is defined as information about the quality of work that signals the availability of positive reinforcement for performance improvement. If your feedback is ever perceived as negative, pessimistic, or insulting, it's game over. To reduce variability in the quality plan, BCBAs can use Reid et al.'s (2012) seven-step evidence-based protocol for providing corrective, positive, and optimistic feedback to staff during the analysis step of the quality control cycle. Here are the steps.

Evidence-Based Feedback Protocol Step 1: Initiate Feedback with a Positive or Empathetic Statement

Exactly what form the statement takes should be individualized to the RBT. Examples of initial positive or empathetic statements are, "I noticed you not only prompted errorlessly, but were able to fade from a partial physical prompt to a gestural prompt and that was impressive", "Her hitting and pinching can be very difficult to ignore and I think you did a great job", or "I know you were nervous about implementing this new protocol with me observing today, but you jumped right in anyway. As a result, we learned something important about this intervention".

Evidence-Based Feedback Protocol Step 2: Make Statements About Behavioral Intervention Protocol Steps or Data Collection Procedures Implemented Correctly

Try to avoid general statements such as "nice work", "good job", or "that went well". Be specific about exactly what the RBT did that aligned with the quality plan, as illustrated in the examples above. In addition to the advice from Reid et al. (2012), I recommend also making an optimistic statement at this step about opportunities to improve performance before specifying what the RBT performed incorrectly. A quick well-timed statement about one or more deviations from the quality plan that represent opportunities to improve implementation in the subsequent cycle may increase the likelihood that the corrective feedback functions as a discriminative stimulus for positive reinforcement in the form of the opportunity to immediately engage in another quality cycle and demonstrate improved performance for the BCBA supervisor. It is as simple as saying, "I noticed something we can improve to help your client learn faster".

Evidence-Based Feedback Protocol Step 3: Tell the RBT What They Performed Incorrectly, If Applicable

After providing both positive and empathetic feedback, and making an optimistic statement about improvement, the BCBA should explicitly tell the RBT about any errors of omission (i.e., steps of the protocol not implemented) or commission (steps implemented that are not in the protocol) noted during the observation, behaviors the client did or did not engage in that might underlie differences in interobserver agreement, or both. For example, "the intervention calls for maintaining continuous attention as you take turns with the toy, but I noticed that you withheld attention on each trial", or "each high-probability response should be reinforced to increase the likelihood the learner will comply with the low-probability response. I noticed you only reinforced low-probability responses". In addition to the recommendation from Reid et al. (2012), I recommend also asking the RBT if they think you missed something in your observation, because in some cases, you will!

Evidence-Based Feedback Protocol Step 4: Tell the RBT What They Should Do to Improve the Quality Plan in the Next Cycle

After telling the RBT that there is an opportunity for improvement, and which step was performed incorrectly, immediately state what they can do differently to implement the quality plan in the next quality control cycle. Reid et al. (2012) warn that your RBT can quickly become frustrated if you give feedback on their performance errors but are unable to tell the RBT how to improve because you lack mastery of the relevant concepts and skills yourself. For advanced RBTs or perhaps BCBA-RBT dyads who are fluent in quality control, it may benefit the dyad if the BCBA instead asks the RBT what they think could be done to implement the quality plan as long as the BCBA rescues the RBT if they don't have suggestions. In addition to recommendations from Reid et al. (2012), I would recommend encouraging the RBT to challenge your feedback and evaluate whether your suggestion for improving the accurate implementation of the behavioral intervention protocol is in fact correct. In my experience it is very helpful for the BCBA-RBT dyad's relationship and productivity to encourage the RBT to think critically and evaluate your observations, perspective, and recommendations as you deliver feedback because in some instances the BCBA's feedback will of course be incorrect and the RBT will have better ideas.

Skip this step if the RBT performed the behavioral intervention with 100% procedural fidelity or interobserver agreement was 100%. In fact, consider skipping it even if the outcomes are 90%, because other targets may need more of your attention, time and resources.

Evidence-Based Feedback Protocol Step 5: Ask for Feedback From the RBT About the Information Provided

Reid et al. (2012) recommend asking for feedback from the RBT after step four. But as mentioned earlier, in my opinion it is more helpful to solicit feedback and encourage critical thinking from the RBT at steps 3 and 4. The analysis step of the quality control cycle is supposed to be very brief. Quality control cycles should be completed quickly. Having something to say but no opportunity to say it can be uncomfortable for an RBT. Every second you can save your RBT from discomfort during the analysis step; it will contribute positively to the overall rate, efficiency, and outcomes of your quality control cycles.

Evidence-Based Feedback Protocol Step 6: Tell the RBT Whether You Want to Conduct Another Quality Control Cycle

Reid et al. (2012) recommended that the BCBA inform the RBT about subsequent supervisory actions. In other words, when they will be observed and receive performance feedback again. However, in contemporary service delivery settings, I believe this is unrealistic. It is really difficult for BCBA supervisors to consistently predict when they will perform any particular supervisory activity because the needs of their clients and clients' families, and the needs of RBTs, can fluctuate unpredictably. A BCBA supervisor who is sensitive and responsive to others' needs will not adhere so strictly to performing activities such a monitoring a specific intervention's implementation at specific days and times determined in advance. In the current model, in this step, the BCBA asks the RBT whether they would like to conduct another quality control cycle on the same target during that same supervision session, and if so, when?

Evidence-Based Feedback Protocol Step 7: Wrap Up the Analysis Step of the Quality Control Cycle with a Positive or Empathetic Statement

In this final step, the BCBA supervisor finishes by again delivering positive feedback, making an empathetic statement, or both. I think Reid et al.'s (2012) advice still applies, but in contemporary ABA practice it is incomplete and outdated. Give a high five or a fist bump! If your RBT is wearing a mask, offer an elbow bump. Give a shout out on your organization's internal electronic communication platform such as Google Chat®. Post something to your colleagues and/or your RBT's colleagues like, "Sarah just crushed a quality control cycle on FCT with client EhCh at 95%! Thanks to Sarah, aggression rates are much lower and we'll be able to start demand fading soon. That's that GOLD STANDARD ABA. Nice work Sarah!".

Evidence-Based Feedback Protocol: Additional Considerations

Successful implementation of this evidence-based protocol requires that the BCBA is competent and fluent in delivering feedback that is also perceived as sincere and maintains privacy (i.e., delivered in private), and functions as compassion. If a contingency that adversely impacts the RBT's response to feedback is discovered, the BCBA should shift their attention away from the outcome of the quality control cycle to eliminating that contingency with compassion (e.g., Melton et al., 2023). For example, if interobserver agreement on a 2D nonidentical matching target is 55%, and data were collected when the client was engaging in particularly high rates of aggression with a known function (attention), the BCBA could take some time to help the RBT implement an abolishing operation, such as fixed-time attention for the aggression, before asking the RBT to implement the next quality control cycle.

RBT Response to Feedback

The BCBA feedback that is corrective or affirming, positive, optimistic, and compassionate, has the potential to improve and maintain RBT implementation of behavioral interventions through quality control cycles. The feedback is delivered in the analysis step of the quality control cycle. The feedback provided to the RBT during the analysis step of one cycle can determine the RBT's implementation of the quality plan in the subsequent cycle. Thus, variation in the extent to which RBTs reinforce or punish BCBA feedback delivery can contribute to variability in quality control frequency, efficiency, and outcomes. To control for this source of variability, preliminary research (Erlich et al., 2023) suggests that BCBAs can help their RBTs acquire a repertoire for responding to BCBA feedback in a manner that reinforces effective and appropriate feedback.

Erlich et al. (2023) reviewed relevant literature and interviewed high-level ABA practitioners and owners of organizations about their preferences for how staff behave in response to feedback in the workplace. Based on the information gathered, they identified eight target skills that comprise a potential repertoire of responding to feedback that could be both highly desirable by supervisors and managers in ABA autism service organization settings, and reinforcing for practitioners who are tasked with providing staff with feedback on a daily basis.

Arrives Prepared for the Meeting

The authors reasoned that "being prepared (e.g., having a writing utensil and notepad) enables a written record of the feedback and the ability to document specific steps for correction" (p. 22). In a quality control cycle, this means that the RBT has participated in the preceding steps of the quality control cycle and may also have something to take notes on in response to the BCBA's feedback. However, in most instances of quality control cycles, RBTs will not write down the BCBA's feedback. At least not in the current model. In the current model the RBT is more likely to immediately implement the feedback in the next quality control cycle, or subsequently review written feedback received electronically after the BCBA submits documentation of the outcome of the quality control cycle. Instead, the RBT has a tablet or another data collection device or printed data sheet in hand and is ready to reference the quality plan as they receive feedback and plan to adjust their performance in the next quality control cycle. If the RBT does not have their device or data sheet in hand, or a piece of scratch paper to jot down notes, they may not be ready to receive feedback.

Maintains Eye Contact During the Meeting

The authors explained that "eye contact is an important social cue to indicate to the person giving feedback whether the feedback is being heard" (p. 22). It also signals to the BCBA that reinforcement in the form of responsiveness to feedback is available for feedback delivery, so long as the RBT's response to feedback is reinforcing. If the RBT is looking at the client, organizing materials, or looking away from the BCBA, they may not be ready to reinforce BCBA feedback.

Asks Appropriate Follow-Up Questions

According to Erlich et al. (2023), this "allows [the] employee to obtain additional or clarifying information; enhances quality of feedback" (p. 22). In a quality control cycle, examples of appropriate types of questions include asking about the components of the intervention such as the schedule of reinforcement, prompt fading strategies, discriminative stimuli, instructional materials, requesting clarification on terms and concepts, and how to motivate the client. Nonexamples of follow up questions include the employee asking questions that are unrelated or unclear, or failing to ask for clarification after receiving vague feedback such as "Reinforcer delivery could use some improvement" and the RBT says, "Will do". The RBT responses to feedback incompatible with appropriate follow-up questions include gossip about other employees, defensive statements, statements about who is to blame for the suboptimal quality control cycle outcome, and accusing the BCBA of being biased or unfair in their assessment of the RBT's performance. If the RBT feels that the BCBA's feedback is biased or unfair, they should immediately apologize and adjust their feedback until the RBT is satisfied that feedback is unbiased and fair, then address that concern directly outside of the clinical context. By asking the BCBA appropriate (i.e., on-topic) questions, the RBT initiates collaboration with the BCBA in the analysis of the quality control cycle outcome and problem solving to improve the outcome in the next quality control cycle as needed. This may be especially helpful if there is a large disparity in the behavior analytic verbal repertoires of the BCBA and RBT. If the BCBA uses technical language that the RBT is unfamiliar with, asking follow-up questions can help the BCBA define terms or use more plain language. If the RBT does not ask appropriate follow-up questions when receiving feedback, the BCBA's verbal behavior may not have the intended effects on the RBT's subsequent performance and it might be helpful to model the steps of the behavioral intervention the RBT should perform differently.

Acknowledges Corrective Feedback

When the RBT acknowledges corrective feedback, it "ensures time in [the] feedback session is spent appropriately discussing how to correct mistakes" (Ehrlich et al., 2020, p. 22). In a quality control cycle, the BCBA shares his or her estimate of procedural fidelity or calculated interobserver agreement with the RBT. As they talk about errors or omission or commission observed and make suggestions for how to improve the outcome on the next quality control cycle, the RBT acknowledges that the BCBA provided this information. Examples of acknowledgement include nodding or affirming statements such as "Got it", "I understand", and "okay". Nonexamples are showing unresponsiveness, denying the BCBA's observations, or delaying the end of the cycle or start of the next quality control cycle by trying to explain the mistake.

Active Listening

The RBT "demonstrates feedback was attended to" (Erlich et al., 2023, p. 22) which "allows [the] feedback giver to review the information they've provided" (p. 22). After receiving feedback from the BCBA in the analysis step of the cycle, the RBT briefly summarizes the feedback given. The summary might reinforce the BCBA's feedback delivery but also can help the BCBA detect errors in their feedback. Nonexamples include summarizing the BCBA's feedback incorrectly or not providing a summary of the feedback received.

Commits to Behavior Change

The RBT, "demonstrates that the recipient of the feedback is willing to make the necessary changes to correct the issue" (Erlich et al., 2023, p. 22). For example, the RBT states that they will make the recommended changes in their performance. Nonexamples include expressing a lack of optimism that they can implement the quality plan, and vague responses to the BCBA's feedback such as, "Yeah, ok" or "Alright, thanks". In the analysis step of the quality control cycle, this may take the form of the RBT hearing one or more components of the behavioral intervention protocol they implemented correctly, stating that they will implement those components correctly in the next cycle, and perhaps even asking to jump right into another cycle so they can demonstrate the performance improvement.

Appreciative Statements

Statements of appreciation in response to feedback is thought to, "increase the future probability that the feedback giver will provide corrective feedback again when it is necessary" (Erlich et al., 2023, p. 22). In other words, appreciative statements can reinforce giving corrective or affirmative, positive, and compassionate feedback needed to maintain or improve outcomes in subsequent quality control cycles. Examples include specific statements of appreciation for the feedback such as "That was really helpful feedback", "Thank you for showing me where I can improve", and "I'm confident I know how to meet expectations next time". Nonexamples include vague statements such as "Thanks!" or "I need some time to process that", or no statement of appreciation at all.

Demonstrates Appropriate Overall Demeanor

The RBTs demonstrate appropriate overall demeanor by smiling or expressing interest, leaning into the conversation (literally), and speaking in a friendly tone. Nonexamples include neutral tones, neutral facial expressions, turning away from the BCBA, frowning, crossing arms or slouching, and expressions of resentment or regress. An appropriate demeanor likely functions as an abolishing operation for behaviors the BCBA might otherwise engage in to avoid confrontation or conflict, and perhaps an establishing operation for the BCBA clearly and efficiently giving the RBT the candid feedback they need to hear to improve procedural fidelity or interobserver agreement in the next quality control cycle.

Step 9. Documentation and Progress Monitoring

Very little variability in quality control is likely to be attributable to how you document outcomes of quality control cycles and monitor progress because this step occurs after you have estimated procedural fidelity or calculated interobserver agreement, and collaborated with your RBT on the improvement or lack thereof needed in the next cycle. Variability attributable to this step in the quality control cycle is most likely to reflect typos or errors in data collection. You can reduce variability in outcomes data attributable to documentation and progress monitoring errors by completing quality control cycles at higher rates. As the BCBA or quality manager progress monitors quality control cycle outcomes over time in graphical display (i.e., a dashboard), more data help to reduce the influence of any single data point on the BCBA or quality manager's decision making over time.

Step 10. Repeat Cycles to Meet the Benchmark

In my experience, conducting multiple quality control cycles on the same target within a session almost always produces improvements in BIQ. Improvements in BIQ for a given target can increase the justification to consider that target mastered. However, improvements in BIQ within session resulting from back-to-back quality control cycles do not always maintain between sessions as indicated by quality control checks on the same target in follow up sessions. A failure to maintain high BIQ across sessions can result from BCBAs and RBTs discussing the intervention protocol at the protocol review stage, or when BCBAs and RBTs interact during the implementation and observation period; and this can slow down target mastery. When possible, BCBAs should use between-session variability in BIQ to make informed decisions about when to master targets. If quality control data over time suggest substantial differences in BIQ between sessions for a given RBT or client, the BCBA may want to avoid mastering targets immediately following multiple within-session quality control cycles for individual targets, and master a target only when BIQ is high the first instance of a quality control cycle within-session. The BCBAs who take this approach may worry that they are mastering targets too slowly. But quality control over BIQ is a cultural practice that prioritizes quality over quantity. Don't worry about mastering targets. Focus on mastering targets indicated by high-quality data you can trust. Your clients' wellbeing depends on it. To accelerate target mastery, avoid discussing the intervention protocol during the review step or interacting with the RBT during implementation and observation.

Chapter Summary

Troubleshooting barriers at each step of the quality control cycle can reduce variability in the incidence and outcomes of quality control over BIQ and BCBA-RBT dyad resistance to managing BIQ. In step one, increases in the initiation of quality control cycles can be achieved with a job aide for cycle starter phrases the BCBA can use to initiate quality control cycles, by setting alarms on data collection devices such as tablets or phones, with session checklists, with prompts from quality managers via internal group chat applications, using delays to BCBA feedback during supervision sessions, and by conducting remote micro-supervision sessions.

In step two, variability in BIQ can be reduced by strategically selecting targets based on the RBT's prior exposure or familiarity with a target before conducting a quality control cycle.

In step three, BCBAs can reduce variability in implementation of the quality plan by standardizing how protocols are written, ensuring the RBT and BCBA independently review the protocol in advance, by correcting obvious mistakes in the protocol, and by withholding discussion of the protocol before selecting procedural fidelity or interobserver agreement as the focus of the quality control cycle.

The decision to focus on dependent or independent variable quality in step four can influence variability in quality control cycle incidence and BIQ (i.e., quality control outcomes). For some dyads, interspersing multiple cycles to assess dependent variable quality between assessments of independent variable quality might increase the rate at which BCBA-RBT dyads conduct quality control cycles.

In step five, variability in quality control cycle incidence and BIQ can be controlled by making sure you define the observation period (e.g., the number of trials or duration of observation) in a manner that results in a representative sample of the overall procedural fidelity or interobserver agreement for a given target and for the client's treatment plan overall. In general, more trials and longer observation periods can be expected to yield more representative data.

In step six, variability can be controlled by helping the RBT to implement the protocol under motivationally optimal conditions for their client.

During step seven, BCBAs should avoid interacting with the RBT or the client to ensure they do not introduce extraneous variables into the environment that influence the RBT's implementation of the protocol. Talking to the RBT or the client during the observation period could evoke or abate behaviors from the RBT or client that do not originate with the behavioral intervention protocol and therefore mislead the BCBA to believe the protocol has effects on the RBTs performance that it in fact does not have. Additionally, the BCBA may fail to notice critical changes in how the protocol is written to ensure that the RBT will implement the protocol with high procedural fidelity and interobserver agreement when the BCBA is absent.

For step eight, this chapter describes research supported steps that BCBAs can take to effectively deliver corrective or affirming, optimistic, and positive feedback to RBTs to maintain or increase BIQ in subsequent quality control cycles, as well as how RBTs can respond to feedback to benefit from the feedback through improvements in performance and reinforce BCBA feedback delivery. BCBAs are encouraged to monitor data-collection accuracy in step nine to reduce variability in documented BIQ due to data-entry errors. For step ten, BCBAs are encouraged to prioritize quality over quantity by noticing when the outcomes of quality control cycles do not maintain across sessions and consider only mastering targets when the first quality control cycle on the target in a given session yields high BIQ.

References

Carr, E. G., & Durand, V. M. (1985). Reducing behavior problems through functional communication training. *Journal of Applied Behavior Analysis, 18*, 111–126. https://doi.org/10.1901/jaba.1985.18-111

Daniels, A. C., & Daniels, J. E. (2006). *Performance management.* Performance Management Publications.

Ehrlich, R. J., Nosik, M. R., Carr, J. E., & Wine, B. (2020). Teaching employees how to receive feedback: A preliminary investigation. *Journal of Organizational Behavior Management, 40*, 19–29. https://doi.org/10.1080/01608061.2020.1746470

Greer, R. D., & McDonough, S. H. (1999). Is the learn unit a fundamental measure of pedagogy? *The Behavior Analyst, 22*, 5–16. https://doi.org/10.1007/BF03391973

Linnehan, A. M., Abdel-Jalil, A., Klick, S., Amey, J., Yeich, R., & Hetzel, K. (2023). Foundations of preemptive compassion: A behavioral concept analysis of compulsion, consent, and assent. *Behavior Analysis in Practice.* https://doi.org/10.1007/s40617-023-00890-1

Mace, C. F., Hock, M. L., Lalli, J. S., West, B. J., Belfiore, P., Pinter, E., & Brown, D. K. (1988). Behavioral momentum in the treatment of noncompliance. *Journal of Applied Behavior Analysis, 21*, 123–141. https://doi.org/10.1901/jaba.1988.21-123

Melton, B., O'Connell-Sussman, E., Lord, J., & Weiss, M. J. (2023). Empathy and compassion as the radical behaviorist views it: A conceptual analysis. *Behavior Analysis in Practice.* https://doi.org/10.1007/s40617-023-00783-3

Michael, J. L. (2004). *Concepts & principles of behavior analysis* (revised ed.). Association for Behavior Analysis International.

Reid, D. H., Parsons, M. B., & Green, C. W. (2012). The supervisor's guidebook: Evidence-based strategies for promoting work quality and enjoyment among human service staff: Vol. 5. *The behavior analysis applications in developmental disabilities series.* Habilitative Management Consultants, Inc.

Silbaugh, B. C., Swinnea, S., & Falcomata, T. S. (2018). Clinical evaluation of physical guidance procedures in the treatment of food selectivity. *Behavioral Interventions, 33*(4), 403–413. https://doi.org/10.1002/bin.1645

The Council of Autism Service Providers. (n.d.). *Practice parameters for telehealth ABA.* https://www.casproviders.org/practice-parameters-for-telehealth##

7 Next Steps

If you did NOT master quality control over behavioral interventions YET, return to chapter six. Please do not give up. I believe any BCBA can master the practices described in this handbook and every bit of effort you put into it will pay off.

If you have mastered quality control over behavioral interventions, or you are a non-clinical member of the ABA autism services macrosystem, proceed with this chapter!

The methods in this book, if implemented consistently by practitioners, can have a profoundly positive influence on their entire organization and every family or student the organization serves. But there is a whole lot more to high-quality ABA service delivery than attaining high BIQ conceptualized as high procedural fidelity and interobserver agreement over time. This chapter only marks the end of the beginning of your new quality assurance journey. There is a long journey ahead and it will look different for everyone. If you are not a behavior analyst in clinical practice, do not worry, keep reading. There is something here for you too!

My Journey in Quality Control Over BIQ

I practiced as a BCBA in ABA autism service delivery for ten years before I developed the practices in this book. As a researcher, assessing procedural fidelity and interobserver agreement were routine practice. But as a practitioner, I rarely assessed procedural fidelity or interobserver agreement. It's not because I didn't care (obviously!) or I didn't work hard. I suggest it's because in clinical practice there are just too many contingencies competing for your attention to assess procedural fidelity with any regular frequency using the methods that textbooks (and for some of us, research training) taught us—trial-by-trial observation and monitoring of each individual component of the behavioral intervention, with a data sheet individualized to the intervention.

In 2022, I had the pleasure of working remotely for Dr. Robbie El Fattal, CEO of Maraca Learning, to help establish Maraca and its first clinic in Boise, Idaho. One of my responsibilities was to develop Maraca's initial RBT

DOI: 10.4324/9781003475095-7

training program to enable new-hire behavior technicians to meet requirements to sit for the RBT certification exam. At the time, the Autism Partnership Foundation, the home of "Progressive ABA", offered a free online 40-hour RBT course that any organization could use to train their RBTs. I sat through the entire course to familiarize myself with the content, evaluate its suitability for Maraca, and develop our RBT training program. While watching a video in one of the course units, I discovered their estimation method for collecting data during discrete trial training (Ferguson et al., 2020).

Best practices in ABA for progress monitoring behavior change and evaluating the effects of behavioral intervention include direct observation and measurement of behavior when the conditions in which the methods are used, allow it. Methods of direct continuous measurement of behavior such as frequency, latency, and duration recording, are common practice. For example, for the purpose of evaluating the effects of an intervention to replace tantrums with communication, we can repeatedly measure frequency, latency, or duration of tantrums over time which enable us to make data-based decisions until we achieve the desired behavior change. Similarly, behavior analysts can manage RBT performance by progress monitoring their mastery of certain best practices in behavioral intervention. For instance, in protocols written for mand training, the BCBA can use direct continuous measurement to monitor the RBT's correct implementation of mand training with a frequency count of the number of steps implemented correctly during an observation period, and calculate the percentage of steps implemented correctly.

Ferguson et al. (2020) point out that in practice, continuous measurement procedures can be difficult to implement consistently with clients. For example, it may not be feasible to use continuous measurement procedures for long periods of time, sometimes a separate observer is needed, high rates of behavior are difficult to measure accurately and consistently, demands are placed on the observer to collect data on many different behaviors, and direct continuous measurement can disrupt the ongoing therapy session because it is hard to maintain engagement with a client when you have to look away from the client, look at a tablet, and collect a data point, for every trial.

These barriers apply to monitoring RBT performance too. In the assessment of procedural fidelity, direct continuous measurement of RBT performance may not be feasible for long periods of time. Sometimes another observer is needed to rule out bias in measurement by the observer. The natural pace of the RBT's target protocol implementation may be too fast to measure accurately and consistently without video recording and reviewing the video later. The BCBAs have to pay attention to many aspects of the clinical environment while observing the RBT implement protocols, and collecting data on every component of a behavioral intervention implemented by the RBT each trial requires that the BCBA frequently look away from the RBT and client to collect the data. Additionally, it often requires that the BCBA have access to a data sheet sufficiently individualized to adequately capture the unique components of the target behavioral intervention.

In an extension of research conducted by Taubman et al. (2013), Ferguson and colleagues (2020) conducted an experimental evaluation with single-subject design methodology to compare trial-by-trial data collection and an estimation method of data collection in teaching expressive labels to children with autism. The study aimed to better understand the extent to which estimation data collection (a) matched trial-by-trial data collection in terms of accuracy, (b) was sufficiently sensitive to target mastery, and (c) teaching was more or less efficient between trial-by-trial and estimation data collection. The authors conducted the study in a clinic and the participants were a 5-year-old boy, and 6-year-old boy, and a 6-year-old girl with autism and Vineland-3 adaptive composite scores between 83 and 85. Pencil and paper data sheets were used to collect trial-by-trial data. For each trial within a session, the interventionist circled one of the following based on the learner's response: "-", "NR", "P+", "P-", or "+", with minus and plus indicating incorrect or correct respectively, "NR" meaning no responses, and "P+" and "P-" meaning successful or unsuccessful prompt, respectively. Estimation data were collected on a 0–4 scale. At the end of each session, the therapist scored 0 if the child responded correctly for 0–20% of trials, 1 for 21–40% of trials, 2 for 41–60% of trials, 3 for 61–80%, and 4 for 81–100% of trials. All sessions were video recorded so the researchers could make comparisons between data-collection methods. Of the 28 sessions that the interventionist used the estimation method of data collection, when compared to trial-by-trial data collection, 27 of the sessions were considered accurate. No differences in the average number of trials ran per session between the estimation method and trial-by-trial method were observed, suggesting in this particular study, the estimation method was not more efficient. It is notable however that sessions were only three minutes in duration. The estimation method may produce more efficient teaching during longer periods of implementation because more time can be spent engaged with the client, especially with a fast pace of trials. In plain language, the estimation method was sufficient for progress monitoring and data-based decision making, and it was sufficiently accurate to determine mastery.

Post-Maraca, I began working for New Beginnings Academy as a full-time clinical supervisor. And it occurred to me that the very efficient and practical estimation method of data collection for discrete trial training might also be a very efficient and practical method for assessing procedural fidelity, and perhaps could help me balance procedural fidelity assessment with everything else that my position required of me. I would just estimate the RBT's behavior instead of the learner's behavior! After all, I did not need precision because if procedural fidelity or interobserver agreement fall below 90%, improvement is needed. It does not matter if procedural fidelity assessment precision is lacking because regardless of whether the outcome is 60% accurate or 80% accurate, it still needs improvement. What was more important than the precision of my procedural fidelity and interobserver agreement assessments, was the rate at which I engaged in these practices. I knew that to teach my RBTs to independently read my protocols and implement interventions accurately over time, collect valid learner data over time that were sufficient to inform my treatment decisions, and enable a relatively high rate of the clinical practice to maintain over time, we would need a method that allows us to engage in the practice frequently despite competing demands placed on us. Perhaps, sometimes taking precedent over everything else I do as a clinical supervisor. I also believed that the high rate of engaging in quality control cycles across a wide variety of behavioral intervention protocols would serve as multiple exemplar training for my RBTs and result in a generalized behavioral intervention implementation repertoire.

I think that the ability of an RBT to read any behavioral intervention protocol and implement it with no further questions at 90% procedural fidelity is the holy grail of RBT training. Early into the development of the current model for quality control, I attended monthly meetings with colleagues at the Michigan Behavior Analysis Providers Association Quality Committee. It was through the committee I met my friend and colleague, National Director of Clinical Quality at Acorn Health, Paul Doher. Paul and I would periodically get together via videoconference in the evenings for a "whiskey zoom" to have a drink and talk ABA, especially ABA quality. In my conversations with Paul, I learned that standardizing the format and terms we use to write our behavioral intervention protocols might help further reduce variability in procedural fidelity. Specifically, I believed that as long as I wrote behavioral intervention protocols in a consistent format, through differential reinforcement of correctly reading and implementing the protocols my RBTs would learn to implement any behavioral intervention protocol in the future with 90% accuracy, even if the interventions I write do not produce desired behavior change. Of course, we want our interventions to produce the desired behavior change from the outset, but quite often we need to evaluate multiple manipulations of independent variables over time. In order to produce the desired outcome, the process requires that protocols are implemented correctly and consistently every step of the way (i.e., in every phase of the evaluation), even when the data show the current phase of the intervention is not working.

My quality control journey continues. As I write this book, I continue to refine the current model of quality control, and engage in both research and development to better understand the relationship between quality control over behavioral interventions and the quality crisis in the ABA autism services industry. Through a better understanding, I'll continue to capitalize on the circumstances I find myself in to expand the current model beyond BCBA supervision, and further develop processes and systems that occasion and reinforce both quality control over BIQ and other practices that positively impact ASDQ. What will your journey look like?

For the Clinical BCBA

You now have a tool in your toolkit that many, many other professionals in the ABA autism service industry do not. As you spread the word about the benefits of the current model for your practice, and you meet BCBAs and RBTs who have been practicing the old way, I believe Patrick Friman's Circumstances View of behavior will help you to act compassionately to bring your colleagues in contact with this better way to do ABA.

The Circumstances View of Behavior

As Friman (2021) explains, for thousands of years people have focused on the person as the source of their own problem behavior. The assumption is that when someone's behavior is deviant relative to the social norms of a culture, a nearly universal assumption is that their behavior is in fact the result of moral or ethical deficiencies, personality, character, or other traits or states supposedly residing within the individual. This "blame" perspective underlies and is used to justify many forms of harm or mistreatment of others, such as war, domestic violence, and child abuse. The Circumstances View of behavior assumes precisely the opposite. It assumes that behavior is a function of its circumstances. That the explanation for behavior, and the variables that can be modified to change behavior, are in the environment. This view is of course foundational in behavior analysis and you are no doubt more than familiar with it. But I have found that too often behavior analysts have difficulty generalizing the Circumstances View from their clients, to their colleagues, and other stakeholders. I am guilty of it myself from time to time. I think that once you master the current model of quality control over BIQ, you will quickly find that incorporating the process into your practice will produce outcomes of supervision and behavioral intervention that are far superior to how you practiced ABA in the past. When you see colleagues continue to practice the old way, largely assuming and/or ignoring procedural fidelity and interobserver agreement, remember that you were in their shoes once, that their practices are determined by their circumstances, and that they need your help.

For the Parents of Learners with Autism and Related Stakeholders

I hope this book has helped you become a more informed consumer and that you have perhaps used the ideas in this book to advocate for your learner. People with autism have a right to effective behavioral treatment, and you want nothing less for your learner. The BACB's BCBA and RBT ethics codes require we deliver it. Effective behavioral treatment depends on the extent to which practitioners use the evidence-based practice of ABA (Slocum et al., 2014). Even interventions designed consistent with the evidence-based practice of ABA will fail to be effective, or may even cause harm, if BIQ is low.

If you discover that your learner's autism care team fails to regularly (e.g., less than a few times a week) assess procedural fidelity and interobserver agreement, there is a good chance that they do not know how to do it, or their organization has not figured out how to provide them with the time and resources they need to do it. Their training program, mentors, the scientific literature, and safeguards put in place to ensure high-quality service delivery have let them down. Treat them with compassion by helping them advocate for changes in organizational policies, resources, or training they need to implement the practices in this book and increase your learner's access to effective behavioral treatment. You could also offer to help! To the extent that you are involved in your learner's ABA therapy, you too can participate in quality control cycles!

For Undergraduate Students Studying Behavior Analysis

If you are an undergraduate student reading this book as a requirement in a course in behavior analysis, consider yourself very lucky. This book is the first of its kind. The field of ABA emerged in the 1960s but ABA service delivery did not really take off until the 1990s to early 2000s. It was not a viable career path, in my opinion, until the early 2000s. The first RBTs were certified by the BACB in 2014. Prior to the publication of this text, I think it is safe to say almost nobody who took an undergraduate course in behavior analysis learned anything about quality control over behavioral intervention! Everyone learns about assessing procedural fidelity and interobserver agreement in their behavior analysis coursework, but very rarely is it discussed exactly how to do those things in practice. This book fills that gap.

When I wrote this book, there were over 160,000 RBT certificants according to the BACB's Certificant Data (BACB, 2024). With the exception of my RBTs, and perhaps those of the BCBAs who have attended talks I have given on this model since 2023, I believe very few of them read anything about quality control over BIQ in their coursework, or received formal instruction in how to implement quality control cycles. Having learned how to achieve quality control over BIQ, your journey will look much differently than many RBTs and behavior analysts before you. You have a better understanding of the concept of quality as it pertains to ABA service delivery (far better than most BCBAs prior to 2024!), the important role quality control over BIQ plays in the bigger picture, and what you can do about it. You will need to put in many years of hard work to become a BCBA and take the lead on quality control in your cases.

If you are an RBT now, or plan to become one, there are steps you can take to increase the likelihood that you work for BCBAs who will provide you with the opportunity to deliver high-quality behavioral interventions. First, make a commitment now to incorporate quality control over behavioral interventions into your practices when you become a BCBA. When you interview for jobs, ask them about the systems and processes in place to ensure you will have the resources needed to deliver effective behavioral interventions, and ask the interviewer to commit to supporting your involvement in quality control over BIQ. If your professor has assigned you the task of learning to participate in quality control cycles with your supervising BCBA, give it everything you have. It is worth it!

If your professor has not given you an assignment to apply the practices in this book, do not let that stop you. Share the book with your BCBAs now. Tell your BCBAs you are committed to nothing less than the implementation of high-quality behavioral interventions in your practice and that the team should start using this model (or a better model if one pops up). Your BCBA may be overwhelmed with a large caseload and it may be hard for them to find the time to listen to your ideas, read this book, and begin engaging in quality control cycles. Assume that they are doing their best and the deck is stacked against them. If they do not control the quality of their interventions, they might be burned out or perhaps recovering from burnout (see Chapter 5). Adopt the Circumstances View of behavior (Friman, 2021), and act compassionately (Melton et al., 2023) by offering to help them eliminate whatever barriers are present that prevent them from engaging in quality control cycles. If you can help them adopt these practices, you might just save their career.

For Graduate Students Seeking BCBA Certification

If you are accumulating fieldwork supervision hours and reading this book as a requirement in a graduate level behavior analysis course, you too, are very lucky. Historically, like undergraduates, graduate students have been taught what procedural fidelity and interobserver agreement are, but not how to implement them with consistency in a real-world practice setting. When you enter into a contract with a BCBA to obtain your supervised fieldwork experience, I recommend starting that relationship by expressing your unwavering commitment to service quality, sharing this book with them, and asking them to help you learn this practice. Researching the literature on procedural fidelity and interobserver agreement assessments, organizing your quality control data, and analyzing quality control data to make data-based decisions about how to increase the rate and outcomes of quality control cycles in your practice will all add to your unrestricted supervision fieldwork experience hours.

Everything you do as an RBT now, and a BCBA in the future, will hinge on whether you can consistently write behavior intervention protocols that RBTs will implement. It will be advantageous to your future work as a BCBA to have experience participating in quality control cycles as an RBT that you can reflect on. Talking about your experience with this process to your future RBTs may motivate them to commit to the process in the same way you have.

Spoiler alert—if you do this, you may discover that the BCBA supervising you does not know how to assess procedural fidelity or interobserver agreement, and in fact may not be able to write behavioral intervention protocols that consistently yield high BIQ. Again, take the Circumstances View. The profession has failed them, but it is not failing you. You and your BCBA now have tools you can use to help yourselves, and the industry, pull out of the quality crisis and deliver a better service. Do not ruminate. Celebrate!

For the BCBA in Operations

In an operations role, you are more concerned with talent acquisition, retaining top talent, client retention, managing schedules, responding to session cancellations, policy implementation, SOAP note quality, and compliance. But my hope is that this book has convinced you that your ability to help your organization operate with excellence depends on assurances that when clients are in direct treatment sessions with their RBTs, the behavioral interventions they receive are the same interventions their BCBAs designed. I hope this book moves you to ask more questions and seek to better understand the role BIQ plays in your clinicians' ability to accept more clients, take on more complex cases, and deliver clinical outcomes that retain clients until they meet discharge criteria.

Please consider sharing what you have learned in this book with your clinical counterpart, such as a clinical director, and starting a discussion about what you can do to help them incorporate quality control over BIQ into their practice. And please consider advocating for your clinical colleagues to leaders in the organization with the power and authority to leverage resources clinical BCBAs need to master quality control over BIQ. Friction between operations and clinical departments is common. If you are in that boat, a shared goal of establishing routine quality control over BIQ, and perhaps working together to understand the relationship between BIQ and employee burnout, might help reduce that friction.

For the Top of the Organizational Chart

If you are a figure at the top of the organizational chart, you are less likely than other members of your organization to have frequent direct contact on the ground with what RBTs and BCBAs do every day. You might be a CEO, a CFO, COO, HR lead, or perhaps even the organization's director of quality! If you hold one of those positions, it is probably very rare for you to spend time observing and directly evaluating how your BCBAs write behavioral intervention protocols and what RBTs do when they read them.

As a result of reading this book, I hope I've opened your eyes to the very real possibility that unless you have designed a system and processes with contingencies that support frequent assessment and remediation of procedural fidelity and interobserver agreement, your BCBAs and RBTs may not be doing their jobs as you expected. It is time to put on your skeptic hat and deep dive into your processing system to determine what is really happening. For more on a systematic approach to designing systems and processes that support high-quality ABA service delivery, I recommend Maria Malott's Culturo-Behavioral Systems (CB-Systems) model of organizational change and engineering because of its compatibility with the ASDQ framework and the science underlying metacontingency control over cultural practices (Malott & Garcia, 1987; Malott, 2003, 2022).

Quality control over BIQ is foundational for quality assurance in ABA autism service organizations. Professionals can build quality assurance from scratch in startup environments. Medium-to-large organizations can redesign or improve quality assurance systems from the top-down (i.e., variability in decision making and resource allocation by leaders high on the organizational chart with power and authority), from the bottom-up (e.g., variability in practices exhibited by clinicians or operators), or a combination of these. A BCBA adopting the quality control practices in this book is an example of a bottom-up approach.

A Bottom-Up Approach

Do your BCBAs already routinely practice quality control over their behavioral interventions? To answer this question, administer a simple in-house survey of BCBAs and RBTs. Administer the survey in-person, such as during a professional development event, to make sure everyone who receives the survey completes it. It might be particularly helpful to ask questions that assess their knowledge of procedural fidelity assessment (e.g., identify the definition, discriminate between examples and nonexamples) and ask them to recall their recent use of these practices. For example, you could ask them to estimate how many times they assessed procedural fidelity last week, and what the outcomes were. Repeated survey administration may provide insights that inform where, when, and with whom you should start observing on the ground and begin collecting baseline data on procedural fidelity and interobserver agreement assessment organization-wide.

Please, prepare yourself for the worst. I am afraid you might not like what you see. But rest assured, if probes of procedural fidelity and interobserver agreement throughout your organization are infrequent, reveal large gaps between what protocols say and what RBTs do, or both, this is not a disaster. It is an absolutely fantastic opportunity to get at the root cause of many of your organization's internal problems, identify a root cause of your organization's own "quality crisis", and to lead your people out of it.

Put together a team consisting of your top performing clinical director, one or two top performing clinical BCBAs with a strong record of leadership, and three or four of their top performing RBTs. Then give them this book, offer them all the resources you have to spare and your unwavering commitment to ensure their success, and give them three to six months to perfect the practice. If quality control does not become a prominent practice for this cohort, determine what the barriers are and remove them. And consider trying again with another cohort. Do not stop until every clinician in your organization controls BIQ. Their ethical code requires it, and your organization's ability to deliver on its promise to customers depends on it.

A Top-Down Approach

I hope one of your next steps is to rally your colleagues and instigate improvement in quality assurance from the top down with the ASDQ framework (Silbaugh & El Fattal, 2021; Silbaugh, 2022; Townsend et al., 2023). An organization demonstrates high-quality ABA autism services in an ASDQ framework to the extent that it attains its own professional and consumer standards with strong financial health over time. High-quality ABA autism services in combination with other services the autism population receives in a broader sense can enhance care quality, or, "The degree to which health services for individuals and populations increase the likelihood of desired health outcomes and are consistent with current professional knowledge" (IOM, 1990a, p. 21). Potential advantages of adopting an ASDQ framework include avoiding prioritizing profit over quality, the ability to coherently integrate professional and consumer standards from multiple sources, a focus on the contingencies controlling quality within the organization; and the ability to adjust professional and consumer standards, corresponding benchmarks, and varying cultural practices adaptively when organizations encounter changes in the conditions under which they operate (Silbaugh & El Fattal, 2021). Silbaugh and El Fattal (2021) issued a five-step call to action with steps leaders can take in a top-down approach to quality assurance with an ASDQ framework: (1) engage in strategic planning with a focus on quality, (2) link strategic initiatives to quality indicators on an internal dashboard to help leaders make decisions that support quality, (3) develop standards and benchmarks for performance and financial health indicated by quality dependent key performance indicators, (4) arrange contingencies that promote operational and clinical quality growth, and (5) publicly report ASDQ metrics. Top-down implementation of an ASDQ framework for quality assurance with these action steps will require considerable leadership, especially in medium and large ABA autism service organizations.

It Will Take Leadership

Building a quality assurance system or convincing others that major improvements in quality assurance are needed, is going to take leadership. But what is leadership? There is no shortage of literature and commercially available books on the topic of leadership, and as anyone with a LinkedIn account knows, no apparent limit in the range of perspectives on what constitutes leadership and who is an expert. There are different kinds of leadership, and they look different depending on the context. For example, President Barack Obama and President Donald Trump demonstrated profoundly powerful leadership. Their leadership during their campaigns was so strong that it got them elected to the presidency. But their leadership styles could not be more different. I am certainly not an expert on leadership. Yet along my own journey I have encountered a few resources that I have found helpful as a behavior analyst working to strengthen the leadership skills needed to establish and disseminate new innovative clinical quality practices within multiple ABA organizations.

One of my favorites is Leading with Gratitude (Gostick & Elton, 2020). Perhaps, because the core ideas in the book align well with my biases: the Circumstances View of behavior and a positive reinforcement approach to building organizational culture. Another book that I think has considerable utility in helping leaders, in ABA organizations in particular, is Aubrey and James Daniels' book "Measure of a Leader" (2005). From the behavior analytic perspective taken in the book, leadership is a process of influencing others, defined and measured in terms of follower behavior.

The authors identify four characteristics of follower behavior that define the effects of leadership. First, followers produce discretionary behavior that directly impacts the leader's goals. These are employees who go the extra mile without being asked to, and for no additional financial compensation. They might not even be employees. They may be volunteers or other stakeholders such as board members. As Daniels and Daniels explain, "The leader's function is to give as many people as possible a cause that transcends their financial involvement" (p. 22). Second, followers sacrifice things like time, resources, authority, or responsibility for the leader's cause. The follower exhibits a commitment to the leader's cause entirely in the absence of pressure, coaxing, or coercion. Third, followers under leadership influence are more likely to reinforce or correct the behavior of others in relation to the leader's teachings and examples. This is the impact leadership has on relationships among employees and their interpersonal interactions. Fourth, followers try to predict or estimate what the leader would approve or disapprove of and establish guidelines for their own behavior accordingly.

Daniels and Daniels (2005) suggest differences between leaders and great leaders are judged or subjectively evaluated in terms of three criteria: (1) the magnitude of their impact, (2) the duration of their impact, and (3) and the number of followers. In other words, how powerful of an impact do the leader's words have on follower behavior, for how long does that impact last, and how many people are affected. Strong leaders are often recognized for having significantly expanded the enterprise, enabled the enterprise to achieve a level of prominence, and left the enterprise with a positive legacy. We can think of magnitude, duration, and the number of followers as indicators of the strength of the influence of the leader on followers, or of the "leader-follower" relation.

Becoming a more effective leader then means effectively strengthening functional relations between your behavior in an organization and the behavior of those whom might become your followers. Strengthening the evocative effects of your behavior on the behavior of others down the organizational chart. Measurement of leader-follower relations is essential if you want to systematically and effectively acquire and improve on your leadership skills, and their effects on organizational culture. Each of the four characteristics of follower behavior can be conceptualized slightly differently in a way that is more conducive to measurement.

Daniels and Daniels (2005) list and describe four categories comprising 12 dependent variables or key performance indicators of leader-follower relations: momentum, commitment, initiative, and reciprocity. The 12 key performance indicators are mass, velocity, direction (for momentum), vision, values, and persistence (for commitment), teamwork, interfaces, and innovation (for initiative) and trust, respect, and growth (for reciprocity). The authors explain that these indicators are far more useful than the more common enterprise growth, enterprise prominence, and legacy indicators because they yield predictive and objective data the leader uses on a daily basis to improve and strengthen leader-follower relations and their effects on the culture and organizational health.

Through radical behaviorist and functional contextualist lenses, leadership is a functional relation between the leading behavior of someone with followers and the behavior of those followers whom the leader has influence over. Someone in the leading role of a leadership relation with followers in an organization engages in behavior that increases the likelihood that other members of the organization follow the leader's compass (i.e., share and believe in their vision), share the same core organizational values, and emulate the leader's behavior as it relates to the cultural practices reinforced by those values. If the organization sets benchmarks for processes, procedures, and practices needed to yield high-quality services, and the leaders' behavior directly influences reductions in variability and waste, helping members of the organization to achieve the quality benchmarks, this is an indicator that leadership is strong. If everything you do in an organization is focused on quality, and you are a leader, the strength of your leadership is the extent to which other members of the organization too will focus on quality in many of the same ways. Leaders lead because followers follow. Their behaviors are interlocked. Followers reinforce the leader's behavior. Leading (i.e., engaging in leader behavior) in a leadership relation is therefore operant behavior shaped by consequences mediated by its followers. It follows that leading is a skill that can be practiced and mastered. Are you a leader? If the answer is no, I encourage you to respond differently next time with "not yet!".

Note that leadership in an organization is a whole lot more than other members of the organization imitating you. It is bigger than that. I do not believe it is enough to model cultural practices you want to see in your organization and motivate people with your words (although that is important too, as discussed later with the "value proposition"). I believe a large part of being an effective leader of cultural change needed to improve ASDQ in an organization is identifying and describing the cultural practices needed to yield high-quality ABA services, describing the context in which those practices can occur, and then through analysis and engineering processes successfully predicting and influencing the cultural practices needed to meet quality benchmarks and consistently deliver high-quality services. If you have influence over a large proportion of an organization's members, and the strength of the leader-follower relation is strong, but you fail to ensure direct relations between follower behavior and service quality, your leadership on quality is ineffective.

All of this goes to say that it appears useful empirically to define leadership in terms of the behavior of the follower, and to assume that (a) there is no one leadership style, (b) leadership is occasioned and reinforced, and (c) leadership behaviors vary within and across contexts. Krapfl and Kruja (2018) described 10 characteristics of a broadly applicable leadership repertoire you can use to guide the self-assessment of your current leadership repertoire and help you focus on the skills you may need to practice and master for the purpose of more effectively leading on quality assurance initiatives from the bottom-up and the top-down.

According to the authors, leaders make a strong value proposition; behave ethically; make things happen; they are innovative; and their communication is clear, concise, direct, and includes the big picture. They improve employee performance not through aversive control but by providing conditions at work that help others grow. They assemble highly effective teams by bringing people of diverse backgrounds and experiences together and putting the right people in the right seats. They confront adversity and solve complex problems by being constantly optimistic, frequently monitoring progress, and developing frameworks they can use to solve new complex problems. When things do not go according to plan, leaders persist. And leaders build a culture that quickly addresses employee underperformance or the shirking of responsibilities and also secures the support of others who can compensate for gaps in the leader's repertoire. The value proposition is foundational to all the rest.

Krapfl and Kruja (2018) explain that a value proposition is a leader's verbal behavior about the potential functional relation between the reinforcing effects of a service or product for the consumer and the reinforcement employees will experience as a result of providing the service or product.

The language of the value proposition contrasts the organization's products and services against its competitors as more reinforcing. Value propositions, which may be implicit or explicit, also give employees clear expectations of what the performance underlying the service or products should look like, and reinforcement they can expect to contact as a result of the performance. In other words, value propositions establish motivating operations and discriminative stimuli in the workplace needed to occasion employee performances that deliver reinforcing products and services for consumers and employees. I will leave you with bottom-up and top-down value propositions to help you get started now.

A Bottom-Up Value Proposition

Here is a value proposition for your *bottom-up approach* you can use to begin leading the adoption of the practices in this book: Tell your colleagues and employees that you believe high-quality behavioral intervention increases the likelihood of the kinds of behavior change in clients that will reinforce consumers' decisions to continue seeking services from our organization. Or, "I believe quality control over BIQ will make our services more valuable to consumers". Then tell them that high BIQ can be achieved consistently with processes that reinforce the clinical cultural practice of frequently assessing procedural fidelity and interobserver agreement. Or, "We can achieve quality control over BIQ by making it a top priority in our clinical system". Then tell them that consumer satisfaction and desired client behavior change resulting from interventions delivered with high BIQ will reinforce our staff's continued implementation of behavioral interventions with high BIQ. Or, "Returns on investment will include increased consumer loyalty and retention of top talent".

A Top-Down Value Proposition

Here is a value proposition you can use in your *top-down approach* to improving quality assurance with the ASDQ framework: Tell them that you believe high-quality ABA service delivery quality defined in terms of standards attainment and communicated with corresponding quality metrics will help your organization adapt and thrive in an ABA autism servicemacrosystem selective for care value. Or, "We can continue to secure insurance authorizations and re-authorizations for services in the future when they begin to require that we report on the quality of our services in combination with clinical outcomes". Or, "Our payors will continue to value our services in the market of the future which will require us to compete with other organizations on quality". Then tell them that high-quality ABA services can be delivered consistently with the implementation of an ASDQ framework which includes strategic planning to link financial goals with quality goals using quality-dependent key performance indicators, using dashboards to frequently monitor standards attainment and engage in continuous improvement, designing systems and processes comprised of reinforcing contingencies that support high-quality service delivery over time, and publicly reporting our quality metrics and soliciting reinforcing feedback from those stakeholders. Or, "We can build an organization that consistently delivers high-quality services by making quality, not quantity, our top priority". Then tell them that high-quality ABA service delivery in an ASDQ framework will improve your competitiveness and help you build an adaptive organization that continues to grow and thrive in changing markets indefinitely. Or, "This approach will help us maintain the demand for our services over the long-term without losing sight of our mission, vision, and values".

For Professors

Imagine every student in your courses accumulating field experience supervision hours, passing all their ABA courses, passing the certification exam, and providing ABA services to the children with autism in your neighborhood, and having no standardized process or data to objectively verify control over whether their behavioral interventions are implemented as designed. The truth is, you do not have to imagine it. It has been happening all along. Chances are that you have watched it happen. Now you can do something about it. You are of course uniquely positioned to influence a new generation of ABA autism service professionals (and probably special educators) to understand and prioritize quality assurance in ABA autism service delivery before they enter the ABA autism services macrosystem as supervising behavior analysts. This is a vital part of your role in your program's quality assurance: making sure practitioners possess the knowledge, skills, and abilities they need to supervise technicians who can implement their interventions with integrity. By assigning this book to your students and teaching them how to implement quality control over their behavioral interventions, you have the power to help many ABA consumers access higher quality care and effective behavioral treatment.

To get you started, I have prepared a sample syllabus for a graduate course in quality control you can add to your verified (and hopefully accredited) course sequence (see Appendix A). I suspect it might fit into your course sequence best, initially, as an elective. But I think training in the current model could be distributed across a semester and interspersed with foundational knowledge in organizational behavior management, so I designed the syllabus to serve as a stand-alone 45-hour course that does just that. Disclaimer: I have not taught the course outlined in the syllabus. I have prepared this sample syllabus so academics can hit the ground running and transfer this information to students as they see fit. You should individualize it to your program and the student population you serve. A tip: To get the most out of such a course, I believe students should actually engage in repeated quality control cycles, analyze their data, and talk about their data and experiences with their classmates. This can be simulated in the classroom first, and subsequently implemented in practice.

For Researchers

There is a long road ahead. Behavior analytic research on ABA service quality, as I write this book, is almost non-existent. This book has laid out but one potential model BCBAs and RBTs everywhere can use now to control the quality of their behavioral interventions. I have found this model to be effective for controlling BIQ in my own practice, but studies should validate the model experimentally. Especially, the estimation method of assessing procedural fidelity, perhaps by comparing estimated procedural fidelity to levels of procedural fidelity obtained with the more rigorous methods historically used in research settings. The current model could be used to experimentally evaluate the variables that control supervision effectiveness over RBT implementation of evidence-based practices in ABA. After working out the variables that influence the occurrence and outcomes of quality control over BIQ, researchers could study the relationship between BIQ and other important aspects of service delivery quality such as clinical outcomes and RBT turnover. There is also a dire need for empirical research on models of quality control over a wide range of other practices common to ABA autism service organizations such as direct treatment session structure, behavioral intervention plan writing, SOAP note writing, discrete trial training, pivotal response teaching, natural environment training, behavioral assessment, functional analysis, BCBA supervision, parent training and related support practices, practices for maintaining customer satisfaction, the process of behavioral intervention implementation (e.g., does RBT visual analysis of graphed data before teaching targets, matter?), RBT training, and more.

Considerably more research is also needed to advance our empirical understanding of ASDQ and variables internal and external to ABA organizations that influence service quality. We need more research to understand whether there is utility in conceptualizing quality at different levels of an organization (i.e., other than at the organizational level), dimensions of quality, relations between the quality of ABA services produced by organizations and cultural evolution phenomena as conceptualized in other disciplines (e.g., tightness-looseness theory), the relationship between quality and access to behavior analysts (which remains inadequate; Yingling et al., 2022), the relationship between quality and outcomes, quality and organizational growth, quality and the structure of organizations, the relationship between quality and leadership, the potential for innovations in machine learning (Lanovaz, 2022) to enhance quality, relations between digital transformation of clinical and operational systems and quality, whether the effects of behavioral interventions (i.e., not just procedural fidelity and interobserver agreement) should be considered when evaluating BIQ, and many more.

Closing

I hope you enjoyed this book and found it useful. If so, please spread the word and you just might help someone else use these practices successfully too. Log in to your favorite social medial platform and post "REAL.QUALITY. CONTROL. -> I have it, and so can you!" with the hashtag "#wedoBIQ" and the link to purchase this book. And tell your audience how the information in this book impacted your practice.

Chapter Summary

This chapter marks the end of the beginning of your journey to support behavioral intervention through routine quality control. My journey continues and so should yours. Clinical BCBA supervisors are advised to adopt the Circumstances View of behavior in supporting their fellow clinical BCBAs in adopting the practice of controlling BIQ with the current model. Parents of learners with autism and other stakeholders are encouraged to use the information in this book as one way to evaluate the quality of their learner's ABA services and potentially support their learner's autism care team by participating in quality control cycles themselves. Undergraduate students in behavior analysis are encouraged to commit to quality control over BIQ and to ask their employers and clinical BCBAs to adopt this model of quality control so that they can best serve their clients as RBTs now and as future BCBAs. Graduate students seeking BCBA certification are encouraged to discuss the current model with their fieldwork supervisor and ask them to incorporate these practices into their training. The BCBAs in operations are encouraged to use the ideas in this book to better understand how quality control over BIQ impacts daily operations, reduce friction between operations and clinical service departments, and work across departments to reduce burnout. This chapter asks individuals at the top of the organizational chart in ABA autism service settings to consider that their practitioners may not control the quality of their behavioral interventions adequately, and to lead initiatives that promote quality assurance from the top-down with the ASDQ framework action steps and from the bottom-up by supporting clinical BCBAs' adoption of the current model. Professors are encouraged to incorporate the current model into graduate coursework in ABA to prepare the practitioners of the future to control the quality of their behavioral interventions. Lastly, researchers are asked to pursue lines of research to help us attain a better empirical understanding of ABA service delivery quality more broadly.

References

Daniels, A. C., & Daniels, J. E. (2005). *Measure of a leaders: An actionable formula for legendary leadership.* Performance Management Publications.

Ferguson, J. L., Milne, C. M., Cihon, J. H., Dotson, A., Leaf, J. B., McEachin, J., & Leaf, R. (2020). An evaluation of estimation data collection to trial-by trial data collection during discrete trial teaching. *Behavioral Interventions, 35*(1), 178–191. https://doi.org/10.1002/bin.1705

Friman, P. C. (2021). There is no such thing as a bad boy: The Circumstances View of problem behavior. *Journal of Applied Behavior Analysis,* 1–18. https://doi.org/10.1002/jaba.816

Gostick, A., & Elton, C. (2020). *Leading with gratitude: Eight leadership practices for extraordinary business results.* Harper Business.

Malott, M. E. (2003). *Paradox of organizational change: Engineering organizations with behavioral systems analysis.* Context Press.

Malott, M. E. (2022). Paradox of organizational change: A selectionist approach to improving complex systems. In R. A. Houmanfar, M. Fryling, & M. P. Alavosius (Eds.), *Applied behavior science in organizations: Consilience of historical and emerging trends in organizational behavior management.* Routledge.

Malott, R. W., & Garcia, M. E. (1987). A goal-directed model for the design of human performance systems. *Journal of Organizational Behavior Management, 9,* 125–129. https://doi.org/10.1300/J075v09n01_09

Melton, B., O'Connell-Sussman, E., Lord, J., & Weiss, M. J. (2023). Empathy and compassion as the radical behaviorist views it: A conceptual analysis. *Behavior Analysis in Practice.* https://doi.org/10.1007/s40617-023-00783-3

Silbaugh, B. C. (2022). Discussion and conceptual analysis of four group contingencies for behavioral process improvement in an ABA service delivery quality framework. *Behavior Analysis in Practice, 16,* 421–436. https://doi.org/10.1007/s40617-022-00750-4

Silbaugh, B. C., & El Fattal, R. (2021). Exploring quality in the applied behavior analysis service delivery industry. *Behavior Analysis in Practice, 15,* 571–590. https://doi.org/10.1007/s40617-021-00627-y

Taubman, M. T., Leaf, R. B., McEachin, J. J., Papovich, S., & Leaf, J. B. (2013). A comparison of data collection techniques used with discrete trial teaching. *Research in Autism Spectrum Disorders, 7,* 1026–1034. https://doi.org/10.1016/j.rasd.2013.05.002

Townsend, D. B., Brothers, K. J., MacDuff, G. S., Freeman, A., Fry, C., Rozenblat, E., DeFeo, D., Budzinska, A., Ruta-Sominka, I., Birkan, B., Hall, L. J., Krantz, P. J., & McClannahan, L. E. (2023). Alliance for scientific autism intervention: System components and outcome data from high-quality service delivery organizations. *Behavior Analysis in Practice.* https://doi.org/10.1007/s40617-023-00898-7

Appendix A
Sample Syllabus

Sample Catalogue Description

ABA XXXX. Intro to Quality Assurance in ABA: Quality Control Over Behavioral Interventions. (3–0) 3 Credit Hours.

Recipients of applied behavior analysis (ABA) services for autism have the right to effective treatment. Effective treatment delivery is also an ethical requirement of behavior analysts. To deliver effective treatment, ABA professionals must deliver high-quality behavioral interventions. Accordingly, this course introduces students to organizational behavior management with a focus on preparing students to engage in ethical and effective ABA practices by collaborating with other practitioners in the delivery of high-quality behavioral interventions in community, in-home, school, or clinic settings. Students learn a brief history of quality, a framework for understanding ABA autism service quality more broadly, and a model for controlling behavioral intervention quality in practice. More specifically, students will apply quality concepts to develop a plan for controlling behavioral intervention quality, implement the plan in practice through service-learning experiences, work together to troubleshoot barriers, and strengthen communication skills by reporting on the outcomes of their quality control practices in class and in a final assignment.

Behavior Analyst Certification Board (BACB) 5th Edition Task List Items

Personnel Supervision and Management—45 Hours

Task List Item	Description
I-1	State the reasons for using behavior-analytic supervision and the potential risks of ineffective supervision (e.g., poor client outcomes, poor supervisee performance).

(*Continued*)

(Continued)

Task List Item	Description
I-2	Establish clear performance expectations for the supervisor and supervisee.
I-3	Select supervision goals based on an assessment of the supervisee's skills.
I-4	Train personnel to competently perform assessment and intervention procedures.
I-5	Use performance monitoring, feedback, and reinforcement systems.
I-6	Use a functional assessment approach (e.g., performance diagnostics) to identify variables affecting personnel performance.
I-7	Use function-based strategies to improve personnel performance.
I-8	Evaluate the effects of supervision (e.g., on client outcomes, on supervisee repertoires)

Purpose and Course Objectives

The purposes of this course are to provide students with a basic understanding of quality assurance in ABA autism service settings, a basic foundation in organizational behavior management concepts and applications, and the skills needed to control the quality of their behavioral interventions in practice, through 45 hours of Organizational Behavior Management coursework to satisfy the 2027 BCBA Pathway 2 Coursework Requirements.

Upon completion of this course, students will be able to

1. Discuss topics in organizational behavior management related to quality assurance in ABA autism service delivery.
2. List major figures and events in the history of managing for quality.
3. Describe and provide examples of quality management, assurance, planning, control, and improvement.
4. Write plans for implementing quality control over behavioral interventions in practice.
5. Describe ABA autism service delivery within the context of the ABA autism service macrosystem and in terms of the metacontingency.
6. Control the quality of behavioral interventions in collaboration with a BCBA clinical supervisor at their practicum, experiential learning site, or place of employment.
7. Troubleshoot barriers to implementing quality control over behavioral interventions.
8. Make systematic clinical decisions in collaboration with a BCBA based on quality control data.
9. Organize, synthesize, analyze, interpret, and present quality control data.

Final Report

The final requirement in this course is the submission of a report containing (a) the student's quality plan, (b) quality control data in graphical form, (c) a summary and interpretation of the data, and (d) a personal reflection on the experience of planning for and controlling behavioral intervention quality.

Recommended Course Schedule

Unit	Topics	Reading Required Before Class	Activities	Test
Unit 1	Course Overview and A Brief History of Quality	Syllabus OBM text or articles Silbaugh Chapter 1	Lecture and small group work	
Unit 2	A Framework for Understanding Quality Assurance	Silbaugh Chapters 1 and 2 OBM text or articles Silbaugh & El Fattal, 2021	Lecture and small group work	
Unit 3	Quality Planning: Part 1	Silbaugh Chapter 2 OBM text or articles Assigned procedural fidelity and IOA articles	Lecture and role-play	
Unit 4	Quality Planning: Part 2	Silbaugh Chapter 2 OBM text or articles	Lecture and role-play	
Unit 5	Logistics and Preparing for Quality Control	Silbaugh Chapter 3 OBM text or articles	Lecture and small group work	
Unit 6	NA	Review Units 1–5 OBM text or articles	Testing on Silbaugh Chapters 1–3 and other articles	Exam 1
Unit 7	Quality Control Week 1 / Cultural Selection	Silbaugh Chapter 4 Culturo-Behavioral Science Metacontingencies OBM text or articles	Lecture and small group work	
Unit 8	Quality Control Week 2 / Management	Silbaugh Chapter 4 Management of quality control cycles OBM text or articles	Brief data-based student presentations on progress Small group discussions and support	

(Continued)

(Continued)

Unit	Topics	Reading Required Before Class	Activities	Test
Unit 9	Quality Control Week 3 / Lab Work	Readings on organizing and analyzing data OBM text or articles	Develop and refine methods for progress monitoring quality control data with Excel	
Unit 10	Quality Control Week 3 / Benefits and Barriers	Silbaugh Chapters 5 & 6 OBM text or articles	Lecture and small group work	
Unit 11	Leading and Other Next Steps	Silbaugh Chapter 7 OBM text or articles	Lecture and small group work	
Unit 12	NA	Review Units 1–5	Testing on Silbaugh chapters 4–7 and other articles	Exam 2
Unit 13	Student presentations	Assigned articles	Discuss outcomes of quality control practices	
Unit 14	Student presentations	Assigned articles	Discuss outcomes of quality control practices	
Unit 15	Student presentations	Assigned articles	Discuss outcomes of quality control practices	Final Report

Author Bio

Bryant Silbaugh, PhD., BCBA, LBA holds a Bachelor of Arts and Master of Arts with majors in Psychology. He received his initial scientific training as a research assistant in behavioral neuropharmacology using operant rodent models at the Scripps Research Institute in La Jolla, California. He received his graduate training in ABA online through the Florida Institute of Technology, and as a doctoral student at the University of Texas at Austin, and subsequently served as an Assistant Professor of Special Education at the University of Texas at San Antonio. Dr. Silbaugh has over 16 years of experience in ABA research, service, and teaching. His research focused on the reinforcement of operant variability, functional communication training, behavioral assessment and treatment of pediatric feeding disorders, and ABA autism service quality. He has published over 20 articles in peer-reviewed journals and a book chapter. Dr. Silbaugh has served as a guest editor for numerous peer-reviewed journals and has given numerous talks on his research at conferences around the country. He is the founder of the National ABA Service Quality Network (NASQN) and continues to conduct research on ABA service quality. Dr. Silbaugh also continues to practice in ABA autism service delivery in a variety of settings.

Index